Reorienting Health Care and Business Sector Investment Priorities Toward Health and Well-Being

PROCEEDINGS OF A WORKSHOP

Theresa M. Wizemann, *Rapporteur*

Roundtable on Population Health Improvement

Board on Population Health and Public Health Practice

Health and Medicine Division

The National Academies of
SCIENCES • ENGINEERING • MEDICINE

THE NATIONAL ACADEMIES PRESS
Washington, DC
www.nap.edu

THE NATIONAL ACADEMIES PRESS   500 Fifth Street, NW   Washington, DC 20001

This activity was supported by contracts between the National Academy of Sciences and the Department of Health and Human Services' Health Resources and Services Administration and Program Support Center, along with Aetna Foundation, The California Endowment, Kaiser Permanente, The Kresge Foundation, New York State Health Foundation, and Robert Wood Johnson Foundation. Any opinions, findings, conclusions, or recommendations expressed in this publication do not necessarily reflect the views of any organization or agency that provided support for the project.

International Standard Book Number-13: 978-0-309-67119-4
International Standard Book Number-10: 0-309-67119-1
Digital Object Identifier: https://doi.org/10.17226/25667

Additional copies of this publication are available from the National Academies Press, 500 Fifth Street, NW, Keck 360, Washington, DC 20001; (800) 624-6242 or (202) 334-3313; http://www.nap.edu.

Copyright 2022 by the National Academy of Sciences. All rights reserved.

Printed in the United States of America

Suggested citation: National Academies of Sciences, Engineering, and Medicine. 2022. *Reorienting health care and business sector investment priorities toward health and well-being: Proceedings of a workshop*. Washington, DC: The National Academies Press. https://doi.org/10.17226/25667.

The National Academies of
SCIENCES · ENGINEERING · MEDICINE

The **National Academy of Sciences** was established in 1863 by an Act of Congress, signed by President Lincoln, as a private, nongovernmental institution to advise the nation on issues related to science and technology. Members are elected by their peers for outstanding contributions to research. Dr. Marcia McNutt is president.

The **National Academy of Engineering** was established in 1964 under the charter of the National Academy of Sciences to bring the practices of engineering to advising the nation. Members are elected by their peers for extraordinary contributions to engineering. Dr. John L. Anderson is president.

The **National Academy of Medicine** (formerly the Institute of Medicine) was established in 1970 under the charter of the National Academy of Sciences to advise the nation on medical and health issues. Members are elected by their peers for distinguished contributions to medicine and health. Dr. Victor J. Dzau is president.

The three Academies work together as the **National Academies of Sciences, Engineering, and Medicine** to provide independent, objective analysis and advice to the nation and conduct other activities to solve complex problems and inform public policy decisions. The National Academies also encourage education and research, recognize outstanding contributions to knowledge, and increase public understanding in matters of science, engineering, and medicine.

Learn more about the National Academies of Sciences, Engineering, and Medicine at **www.nationalacademies.org**.

The National Academies of
SCIENCES · ENGINEERING · MEDICINE

Consensus Study Reports published by the National Academies of Sciences, Engineering, and Medicine document the evidence-based consensus on the study's statement of task by an authoring committee of experts. Reports typically include findings, conclusions, and recommendations based on information gathered by the committee and the committee's deliberations. Each report has been subjected to a rigorous and independent peer-review process and it represents the position of the National Academies on the statement of task.

Proceedings published by the National Academies of Sciences, Engineering, and Medicine chronicle the presentations and discussions at a workshop, symposium, or other event convened by the National Academies. The statements and opinions contained in proceedings are those of the participants and are not endorsed by other participants, the planning committee, or the National Academies.

For information about other products and activities of the National Academies, please visit www.nationalacademies.org/about/whatwedo.

PLANNING COMMITTEE ON REORIENTING HEALTH CARE AND FINANCE SECTOR INVESTMENT PRIORITIES TOWARD HEALTH AND WELL-BEING[1]

BOBBY MILSTEIN (*Chair*), ReThink Health
CATHY BAASE, Michigan Health Improvement Alliance; The Dow Chemical Company
JIM KNICKMAN, New York University
SANNE MAGNAN, HealthPartners Institute; University of Minnesota
LISA RICHTER, Avivar Capital
MYLNN TUFTE, North Dakota Department of Health
CAROLINE WHISTLER, Third Sector Capital Partners

---

[1] The National Academies of Sciences, Engineering, and Medicine's planning committees are solely responsible for organizing the workshop, identifying topics, and choosing speakers. The responsibility for the published Proceedings of a Workshop rests with the workshop rapporteur and the institution.

ROUNDTABLE ON POPULATION HEALTH IMPROVEMENT[1]

SANNE MAGNAN (*Co-Chair*), Senior Fellow, HealthPartners Institute; Adjunct Assistant Professor, University of Minnesota
JOSHUA M. SHARFSTEIN (*Co-Chair*), Associate Dean for Public Health Practice and Training, Johns Hopkins Bloomberg School of Public Health
PHILIP M. ALBERTI, Senior Director, Health Equity Research and Policy, Association of American Medical Colleges
TERRY ALLAN, Health Commissioner, Cuyahoga County Board of Health
JOHN AUERBACH, Executive Director, Trust for America's Health
CATHY BAASE, Chair, Board of Directors, Michigan Health Improvement Alliance; Consultant for Health Strategy, The Dow Chemical Company
DEBBIE I. CHANG, Senior Vice President, Policy and Prevention, Nemours
KATHY GERWIG, Vice President, Employee Safety, Health and Wellness and Environmental Stewardship Officer, Kaiser Permanente
MARTHE GOLD, Senior Scholar in Residence, The New York Academy of Medicine
MARC N. GOUREVITCH, Professor and Chair, Department of Population Health, New York University Grossman School of Medicine, New York University Langone Health
GARTH GRAHAM, President, Aetna Foundation
GARY R. GUNDERSON, Vice President, Wake Forest Baptist Health and Stakeholder Health, Wake Forest University
WAYNE JONAS, Executive Director, H&S Ventures
ROBERT M. KAPLAN, Professor, Stanford University
DAVID A. KINDIG, Professor Emeritus of Population Health Sciences and Emeritus Vice Chancellor for Health Sciences, University of Wisconsin–Madison
PAULA M. LANTZ, Associate Dean for Academic Affairs and Professor of Public Policy, University of Michigan
MICHELLE LARKIN, Associate Vice President and Associate Chief of Staff, Robert Wood Johnson Foundation
THOMAS A. LaVEIST, Professor and Chair, Department of Health Policy, Milken Institute School of Public Health, The George Washington University

---

[1] The National Academies of Sciences, Engineering, and Medicine's forums and roundtables do not issue, review, or approve individual documents. The responsibility for the published Proceedings of a Workshop rests with the workshop rapporteur and the institution.

JEFFREY LEVI, Professor, Milken Institute School of Public Health, The George Washington University
SHARRIE McINTOSH, Vice President for Programs, New York State Health Foundation
ROBERT McLELLAN, Chief, Section of Occupational and Environmental Medicine; Medical Director, Live Well/Work Well; Professor of Medicine, Community and Family Medicine, Geisel School of Medicine at Dartmouth, Dartmouth-Hitchcock Medical Center
PHYLLIS D. MEADOWS, Senior Fellow, Health Program, The Kresge Foundation
BOBBY MILSTEIN, Director, ReThink Health
JOSÉ T. MONTERO, Director, Center for State, Tribal, Local, and Territorial Support; Deputy Director, Centers for Disease Control and Prevention
MARY PITTMAN, President and Chief Executive Officer, Public Health Institute
PAMELA RUSSO, Senior Program Officer, Robert Wood Johnson Foundation
MYLYNN TUFTE, State Health Officer, Office of the Governor, State of North Dakota
HANH CAO YU, Chief Learning Officer, The California Endowment

Health and Medicine Division Staff

ALINA BACIU, Roundtable Director
CARLA ALVARADO, Program Officer (*through January 2021*)
KIMANI HAMILTON-WRAY, Senior Program Assistant (*through May 2019*)
ROSE MARIE MARTINEZ, Senior Board Director, Board on Population Health and Public Health Practice

Consultant

THERESA M. WIZEMANN, Rapporteur

Reviewers

This Proceedings of a Workshop was reviewed in draft form by individuals chosen for their diverse perspectives and technical expertise. The purpose of this independent review is to provide candid and critical comments that will assist the National Academies of Sciences, Engineering, and Medicine in making each published proceedings as sound as possible and to ensure that it meets the institutional standards for quality, objectivity, evidence, and responsiveness to the charge. The review comments and draft manuscript remain confidential to protect the integrity of the process.

We thank the following individuals for their review of this proceedings:

JOSÉ T. MONTERO, Centers for Disease Control and Prevention
MYLYNN TUFTE, North Dakota Department of Health
IVANA VAUGHN, The New York Academy of Medicine
HANH CAO YU, The California Endowment

Although the reviewers listed above provided many constructive comments and suggestions, they were not asked to endorse the content of the proceedings nor did they see the final draft before its release. The review of this proceedings was overseen by **MARTIN J. SEPULVEDA,** IBM Corporation. He was responsible for making certain that an independent examination of this proceedings was carried out in accordance with standards of the National Academies and that all review comments were carefully considered. Responsibility for the final content rests entirely with the rapporteur and the National Academies.

Contents

ACRONYMS AND ABBREVIATIONS   xiii

1 INTRODUCTION   1
Workshop Objectives, 3
Organization of the Workshop and Proceedings, 4

2 CONNECTING HEALTH AND THE ECONOMY: THE SURGEON GENERAL'S CALL TO ACTION   5
Health and the Economy, 5
Discussion, 10

3 EVOLVING VALUES AND PRIORITIES IN HEALTH CARE   11
Shifting Toward New Value and Investment, 11
Engaging Health Systems in Improving Population Health, 13
Aligning Drivers of Accountability and Economic Interest, 14
Taking Action in Health Care, 15
Policy Changes to Consider, 15
Discussion, 16

4 EVOLVING VALUES AND PRIORITIES AMONG BUSINESS INVESTORS   19
Using Capital to Drive Change, 19
Demand Side Perspective: Local Initiatives Support Corporation, 20
Supply Side Perspective: Goldman Sachs, 23

| 5 | **CASE EXAMPLE OF INVESTMENT BY A HEALTH CARE ORGANIZATION** | 27 |

UH: Striving Toward a Culture of Population Health, 27
Discussion, 33

| 6 | **A CASE EXAMPLE OF BUSINESS INVESTMENT** | 37 |

U.S. Trust at Bank of America: Impact Investing, 37
Discussion, 41

| 7 | **REFLECTIONS ON LEADERSHIP INVESTMENT PRIORITIES** | 43 |

Leadership Investment: Small Group Activity, 43
Closing Comments, 50

APPENDIXES
A REFERENCES 55
B WORKSHOP AGENDA 57
C BIOGRAPHICAL SKETCHES 61
D READINGS AND RESOURCES 73
E COMMISSIONED INFOGRAPHIC: PATH TOWARD A WELL-BEING ECONOMY 79
F SMALL GROUP EXERCISE MATERIALS 83

Acronyms and Abbreviations

ACA	Patient Protection and Affordable Care Act
ACO	accountable care organization
CDFI	community development financial institution
CMMI	Center for Medicare & Medicaid Innovation
EHPH	Enhancing the Role of Hospitals in Improving Population Health
ESG	environmental, social, and governance (standards)
LISC	Local Initiatives Support Corporation
NYU	New York University
RWJF	Robert Wood Johnson Foundation
UH	University Hospitals (Cleveland)

1

Introduction[1]

Since 2013, the Roundtable on Population Health Improvement of the National Academies of Sciences, Engineering, and Medicine has been providing a trusted venue for leaders from the public and private sectors to meet and discuss leverage points and opportunities for achieving better population health in the evolving political and social environments, said Sanne Magnan of HealthPartners Institute and the University of Minnesota. The roundtable's vision is of a strong, healthful, and productive society that cultivates human capital and equal opportunity. This vision rests on the recognition that outcomes such as improved life expectancy, quality of life, and health for all are shaped by interdependent social, economic, environmental, genetic, behavioral, and health care factors. Achieving this vision will require national and community-based policies and dependable resources, Magnan continued.

In 1997, David Kindig of the University of Wisconsin–Madison asserted that "population health improvement will not be achieved until appropriate financial incentives are designed for this outcome" (Kindig, 1997, p. 174), and Magnan noted that this statement remains true more

---

[1] This workshop was organized by an independent planning committee whose role was limited to identification of topics and speakers. This proceedings was prepared by the rapporteur as a factual summary of the presentations and discussions that took place at the workshop. Statements, recommendations, and opinions expressed are those of individual presenters and participants and are not necessarily endorsed or verified by the National Academies of Sciences, Engineering, and Medicine, the Health and Medicine Division, or the roundtable, and they should not be construed as reflecting any group consensus.

than two decades later. "We are moving in the right direction," Magnan said, "but with the recent report of declining U.S. life expectancy, there is much more to be done."

The roundtable has considered the topic of resources broadly and from a range of perspectives, and Magnan referred participants to the proceedings of several recent roundtable workshops as examples (see IOM, 2014, 2015a,b; NASEM, 2018, 2019). To further the discussion, on December 3, 2018, the roundtable convened a workshop, hosted by New York University (NYU) Langone Health in New York City, to explore how evolving concepts of value in health care and business investments are leading to a shift in resources toward investments in health and well-being for all. Participants were welcomed by Marc Gourevitch on behalf of NYU Langone Health.

Bobby Milstein of ReThink Health also noted the decades-long history of work on various aspects of the flow of resources for population health. Resources matter, he said, but "to get better results, we must invest differently." New concepts of value and investment have the potential to shift entire sectors of the U.S. economy, Milstein continued. Magnan and Milstein referred participants to an infographic commissioned for the workshop that provides an overview of the ways in which the health care and business investment sectors are moving toward a well-being economy (see Appendix E).

There is both "good news and bad news" along the macroeconomic path to realizing the country's potential for health, well-being, and prosperity, Milstein said. On the negative side, there has been a long history of macroeconomic and market movements (i.e., and their negative effects on workers, communities, and the environment) that have brought us to the realization, stated Milstein, that "until we really bring the value for health and well-being into our markets, we're not going to see the full potential for health and well-being to flourish." On the positive side, investing in health and well-being is now a recognized and visible priority. He mentioned several examples, including emphasis in the forthcoming Healthy People 2030 and the priorities established by the current Surgeon General as well as documents from the Federal Reserve and other financial organizations, on investing for outcomes and value for the long term. There is a movement toward value and an opportunity for leadership, he said. Milstein emphasized leadership opportunities as the focus of the workshop discussions and called on participants to consider what leadership role they could take to drive the necessary investments that will lead to equitable health and well-being.

INTRODUCTION

WORKSHOP OBJECTIVES

The agenda for this workshop was developed by an independent planning committee that included Magnan, Milstein, Cathy Baase (Michigan Health Improvement Alliance and The Dow Chemical Company), James Knickman (NYU), Lisa Richter (Avivar Capital), Mylynn Tufte (North Dakota Department of Health), and Caroline Whistler (Third Sector Capital Partners). (The planning committee's Statement of Task is provided in Box 1-1.) As outlined by Milstein, the workshop objectives were to:

- Reflect on the history and current state of the shift to new values and investment priorities (e.g., living wages or environmental sustainability) within two spotlight sectors: health care and business investments;
- Explore what selected organizational leaders are doing to establish new concepts of value and new investment priorities (including tools and platforms useful to these efforts); and
- Identify leadership and partnership opportunities that could help to further the shift toward new investments that produce equitable health and well-being.

The workshop, a 1-day event, could not include a detailed history of the investment landscape in the business and health sectors, or orient audience members unfamiliar with those fields to the impact invest-

---

BOX 1-1
Planning Committee Statement of Task

An ad hoc committee will plan and convene a 1-day public workshop that will explore some of the factors that can spur change in economic priorities in two spotlight industries: health care and financial services. Both industries are in the midst of a quest to reorient decision making regarding when, where, and with whom to invest resources that affect all lives and livelihoods, and thus shape the conditions for health and well-being. The workshop will feature invited presentations and discussion that will explore (1) the history and current state of the shift to new investment priorities (e.g., environmental sustainability, worker well-being); (2) what industry leaders are doing to make progress and avoid pitfalls; (3) tools and platforms that are useful to these efforts; and (4) lessons and insights that stakeholders can use to help reinforce the shift toward healthier investments. The committee will plan and organize the workshop, select and invite speakers and discussants, and moderate discussions. A proceedings and a proceedings-in-brief of the presentations and discussion at the workshop will be prepared by a designated rapporteur in accordance with institutional guidelines.

ing and community development domains. However, some readings and resources were provided on the workshop web page and by email to registered attendees (see Appendix D), along with a commissioned infographic (see Appendix E), to orient workshop attendees and the broader audience to the topic and to help them enhance their understanding of the subject matter.

ORGANIZATION OF THE WORKSHOP AND PROCEEDINGS

The workshop opened with a keynote address from U.S. Surgeon General Jerome Adams (see Chapter 2). The first two panel sessions of the workshop focused on whole-sector overviews of the evolving values and priorities in health care (see Chapter 3) and in business investments (see Chapter 4). The next two panel sessions provided profiles of selected leaders in the health care (see Chapter 5) and business investment (see Chapter 6) sectors, with attention to how leaders of those institutions reposition their organization's priorities, relationships, and investments in a changing landscape. The workshop concluded with a small group activity that drew from the day's discussions to consider priorities for value and investment, followed by final observations and reflections from Joshua Sharfstein (see Chapter 7). Points of interest were shared on Twitter throughout the day by participants using #pophealthrt.[2]

---

[2] The Twitter discussion that took place on December 3, 2018, in association with the workshop can be viewed at https://twitter.com/hashtag/Pophealthrt (accessed June 23, 2021).

2

Connecting Health and the Economy: The Surgeon General's Call to Action

To open the workshop, Jerome Adams, 20th Surgeon General of the United States and Vice Admiral of the Commissioned Corps of the U.S. Public Health Service, delivered a keynote address issuing a call to action to connect health and the economy. The session was moderated by Cathy Baase of the Michigan Health Improvement Alliance and The Dow Chemical Company. (Highlights of this session are presented in Box 2-1.)

HEALTH AND THE ECONOMY

In defining his priorities as Surgeon General, Adams said he chose to include community health and economic prosperity because he believes those issues have the potential to influence all aspects of health. "Prosperous and economically stable individuals tend to be healthier," he said. At the same time, individuals and communities that are healthier tend to be more prosperous. Adams's signature Call to Action is titled—and will focus on—Community Health and Economic Prosperity, including the role of private-sector investment in promoting community health and economic well-being.[1]

Much of health care, policy, and political debate is focused on optimizing downstream interventions. Adams pointed out, however, that less than 20 percent of health is influenced by health care. Health is influenced

---

[1] For information on the *Surgeon General's Call to Action: Community Health and Prosperity*, see https://www.federalregister.gov/documents/2018/09/06/2018-19313/surgeon-generals-call-to-action-community-health-and-prosperity (accessed June 23, 2021).

> **BOX 2-1**
> **Highlights from the Presentation**
> **by U.S. Surgeon General Jerome Adams***
>
> - The United States lags behind comparable countries in a range of health metrics, and health disparities in the nation are increasing.
> - Addressing upstream determinants of health does not exempt people from personal responsibility, but the choices that people can make are entirely dependent on the choices available to them.
> - Money that individuals and employers must spend on health care is money that could be spent on other priorities, such as education, infrastructure, wage increases, or individual purchases (which stimulate the economy).
> - Healthier people are more productive, and healthier communities are more prosperous and safe.
> - Engaging a broad range of partners to innovate and promote upstream interventions can help communities thrive. Non-traditional partners with community connections can be essential advocates for health in the community.
>
> ---
>
> * This list is the rapporteur's summary of the main points made by Adams and does not reflect any consensus among workshop participants, or endorsement by the National Academies of Sciences, Engineering, and Medicine.

primarily by an individual's environment and behaviors. There is not sufficient investment upstream, he said, in the health and well-being of communities and in activities that could prevent disease and reduce health care costs (e.g., addressing social determinants of health). More value can be obtained from America's health care dollars.

Health in the United States is "far from where it could be," Adams said, and the nation lags behind comparable countries in a range of health metrics. Within the United States, health disparities are increasing. The goal of a healthier, more prosperous, and equitable America cannot be realized unless the upstream determinants of health are addressed, he said. Those determinants of health can provide people with opportunities to make healthier choices. Social determinants of health include, for example, housing, education, employment, transportation, and connections to one's community. These and other social determinants of health "have a profound impact on a person's ability to be born healthy and to stay healthy across the life span, to engage in healthy behaviors, and to avoid conditions like heart disease, diabetes, and obesity," Adams said. Addressing upstream determinants of health does not exempt people from personal responsibility, he continued, but the choices that people can make are entirely dependent on the choices available to them. For example, not all families can choose to send their children outside to play because they may have safety concerns (e.g., traffic, violence). Similarly, many cannot choose to eat fresh fruits and vegetables regularly because grocery stores are less accessible to them than local convenience stores or fast-food restaurants.

Placemaking

Hospitals and health care providers, businesses and employers, and local governments are beginning to recognize the role of a community's environment (i.e., "place") in driving good health, and the role of good health in driving the economic prosperity of the community, Adams said. As an example, he mentioned the recent search by Amazon for a location for a second corporate headquarters. Ultimately, Amazon chose to split its second headquarters between two sites, one in New York City and one in Crystal City, Virginia.[2] Citing *U.S. News & World Report*'s 2018 healthiest communities rankings,[3] Adams suggested that "it's no coincidence" that Crystal City, Virginia, is surrounded by 3 of the top 10 healthiest communities in the country (Falls Church, Loudoun County, and City of Fairfax). While local governments often provide tax incentives to attract businesses, forward-thinking communities are now focused on placemaking. Investing in the health of the community helps to reign in unsustainable health care costs, and Adams added that health care costs for current and future employees is a significant concern for most employers, including Amazon. Every community can become healthier, Adams said, but special attention is needed to address the challenges facing those most in need, in the most disadvantaged communities.

Forging New Partnerships

Adams's motto as Surgeon General, he said, is "better health through better partnerships." The problems that need to be solved are multifactorial and the solutions are complex. The work of improving community health has many stakeholders, and Adams called for forging new, innovative, and broad-ranging partnerships.

Adams spoke about the concept of servant leadership, which he described as "leading by meeting the needs of others, so that their success leads to your success." He said that, as Surgeon General, he is "committed

---

[2] The company announced in February 2019 that it would rescind plans for its New York City location (see, for example, https://www.nytimes.com/2019/02/14/nyregion/amazon-hq2-queens.html [accessed June 23, 2021]).

[3] Available at https://www.usnews.com/news/healthiest-communities/rankings (accessed June 23, 2021).

to being a servant leader, to strengthening connections within the health community, and to forging those new partnerships that can help us solve our most pressing health problems."

As an example of reaching out across silos to forge new partnerships, Adams described engaging the National Association of Attorneys General. Although some might believe the law enforcement community wants only to lock up those suffering from substance use disorder, he said, the fact is that prisons and jails are the largest providers of mental health services in the United States. Potential partners for health can be found in law enforcement, academia, the military, faith leaders, and many other sectors. It is important to invite them to the table as stakeholders in community health, he continued, but also to go to their table, listen, and be a servant leader. Many potential partners, even some in the health sector, are not aware of the value of investing in community health and the potential return on investment, Adams said.

Health care costs account for nearly one-fifth of the U.S. economy, Adams said. Families, businesses, and government all feel the burden of poor health and its impact on prosperity. Currently there are 6 million unfilled jobs in the United States, and Adams noted that many people who might fill these jobs are not looking for work due to health-related issues. Money spent on health care, whether by an employer (e.g., to provide coverage) or an employee (e.g., for a copay or deductible), is money that could be spent on other priorities, he continued. Money not spent on health care could be spent on education, infrastructure, or wage increases, for example, or even on holiday gifts or other purchases that, in turn, stimulate the economy. Adams suggested that a main reason wages have remained stagnant is because businesses are paying higher health care costs.

The outcomes associated with health inequities impact everyone, Adams said. The mission should be to deliver "healthier children to our schools, healthier workers to employers and businesses, and a healthier population to communities," he said. The evidence supports the notion that healthier people are more productive, and healthier communities are more prosperous and safer. Adams noted several examples, including Purpose Built Communities of East Lake, Georgia; Minneapolis, Minnesota, Blue Zones; and Live Well San Diego in California.

The economy has long been a top issue for voters, regardless of party, demographic, or geography, noted Adams. Although many voters in the most recent election cited health care as their top concern, Adams suggested that these voters were not actually voting on health as an issue, but on the economic aspects of health care (i.e., the high costs of health care are impacting their ability to pay for other needs). Education is needed so that employers, policy makers, and the public understand that the return on investment in health is economic development and prosperity for individuals and the community.

Adams said the forthcoming Surgeon General's report will "demonstrate the link between community health and economic prosperity and provide tools for community investment that deliver health impact." These tools can be used by health care organizations, businesses, philanthropies, financial institutions, community planners, and other stakeholders to improve community health and foster prosperity. Adams expressed hope that the forthcoming Surgeon General's report on community health and prosperity will end any debate about the association between health and the economy and will inspire action by all stakeholders in health.

Moving Forward

In closing, Adams reiterated his Surgeon General's Call to Action message to participants, encouraging them to:

- Innovate and promote upstream interventions that can help communities thrive and achieve "better health through better partnerships."
- Engage a broad range of partners in discussions of public health issues, including faith communities, military, local businesses, law enforcement, and others. These stakeholders have influence at the highest policy levels and at critical touch points for community health. Non-traditional partners who have community connections can be essential advocates for health in the community.
- Communicate more effectively that the pathway to prosperous communities starts with healthier communities. Partners in the communities are interested in profits and costs. Focus on how improving health can impact their financial bottom line.
- Incorporate health equity into everything because when health inequity exists, "we all pay the price." Interventions should benefit and be accessible to all communities, and not just improve the health of those who are already doing well. As an example, Adams said there has been success in driving down opioid prescribing rates, but what is often overlooked is the fact that people with unmanaged pain have started using injection drugs instead. Ignoring inequities "makes the problem worse for the communities that are most in need."

"We have the opportunities," Adams concluded, and he said he was ready to work toward improved overall health opportunities and health outcomes for all.

DISCUSSION

In the brief discussion that followed, Joshua Sharfstein of the Bloomberg School of Public Health at Johns Hopkins University asked about incorporating "a constructive discussion on immigration as part of an overall approach to health and the economy." He suggested that current and proposed immigration policies can negatively impact health and observed that immigrants often fill the job vacancies that Adams mentioned. Adams responded that better communication is needed to disseminate the message that "there is a net benefit to making sure there is a reasonable immigration system." A challenge is that one bad story involving an immigrant can taint public perception.

John Auerbach of Trust for America's Health observed that, despite significant attention to obesity as a health issue, the latest data show that obesity rates for both children and adults continue to increase. He asked what could be done differently to see improvement. Adams concurred that addressing obesity in the United States is an ongoing challenge. Better communication is needed about the role of a person's environment in the choices they are able to make, he said, for example, whether they have access to healthy foods, or safe places to be active. Better choices need to be more readily available. There is also a need to create environments that allow people to incorporate being physically active throughout the day, he said, not just when they set aside time to go to the gym.

3

Evolving Values and Priorities in Health Care

For the first panel discussion, Mai Pham of Anthem and James Knickman of the New York University (NYU) Grossman School of Medicine and NYU Wagner Graduate School of Public Service shared their perspectives as leaders in the health care sector about why and how values and priorities are changing in health care. Following the panel discussion, the panelists addressed questions from participants. The session was moderated by Sanne Magnan. (Highlights of this session are presented in Box 3-1.)

SHIFTING TOWARD NEW VALUE AND INVESTMENT

"In health care," Magnan said, "value is often associated with dollars spent for outcomes perceived to have merit or significance." She reiterated the point made by Adams (see Chapter 2) that health care costs continue to increase, and that increased spending on health care often means that funding is being diverted from other priorities (e.g., addressing the social determinants of health). She referred participants to the commissioned infographic, which depicts some of the milestones in the movement by leaders in health care and business investments toward new value and investment in health care (see Appendix E). Magnan emphasized the statement on the infographic that "those shifts are still fragile and incomplete," and asked panelists to comment on why this is the case, to reflect on the milestones, and to suggest other opportunities or milestones to keep pushing toward new value.

> **BOX 3-1**
> **Key Points Made by Individual Speakers***
>
> - Many stakeholders are not yet convinced that the goals of value-based care and population health are also in their own economic self-interest. (Pham)
> - Providers and health systems understand the broader societal community health goals, but respond to the current physician fee schedule. Profit margins for providers vary according to the service, which drives behavior and investments toward income-generating procedures. (Pham)
> - Key drivers of health system investment in community health include engaged leadership; a business case; market competition; multisector partnerships; and public policy and legislation. (Knickman)
> - To prioritize investments, data are needed on the current social circumstances and needs of patients, including qualitative data on the causal pathways that contribute to overall health, and data on which social services are most effective. Robust and integrated data systems and the ability to rapidly evaluate the data are also needed. (Knickman, Pham)
> - From a provider perspective, there are established, evidence-based guidelines for managing prevalent chronic diseases, but there are no comparable guidelines for managing the social determinants of health. (Kaplan)
>
> ---
>
> * This list is the rapporteur's summary of the main points made by individual speakers and participants (noted in parentheses) and does not reflect any consensus among workshop participants, or endorsement by the National Academies of Sciences, Engineering, and Medicine.

Looking back, Knickman said, early milestones that demonstrated a focus on value included the concept of capitation and the creation of health maintenance organizations, such as Kaiser Permanente and others. A more recent milestone was the Patient Protection and Affordable Care Act (ACA). Knickman reminded participants that although there is much emphasis on the coverage aspects for the ACA, it includes important provisions for system transformation. One example is the establishment of the Center for Medicare & Medicaid Innovation (CMMI), which is focused on testing new payment approaches and service models. Knickman also mentioned Delivery System Reform Incentive Payment programs, the Medicaid Innovation Accelerator Program, accountable care organizations (ACOs), health homes, and the Patient-Centered Outcomes Research Institute, which he said have generated momentum and interest. Another key milestone, he said, was the research that "laid the groundwork for understanding the importance of social determinants of health."

Pham added that, early on, the idea that a health care provider should be accountable to a third party or to the public for the quality of care they provided was "revolutionary." She also mentioned the development of measures of quality so that a system of accountability in the marketplace could be implemented. Another "quiet revolution" following the passage of the ACA, she said, was transforming the mindset of care providers from a focus on revenue streams for their practice to an acknowledgment of the need to consider the total cost of care for their patients.

In response to why the transition to value is fragile and incomplete despite the momentum and investment, Pham said that many stakeholders still need to be convinced that the goals of value-based care and population health are also in their own economic self-interest. Knickman agreed and said that the fee-for-service payment model is still dominant. More effective evidence demonstrating the impact of upstream investments is needed to strengthen the transition. He suggested that another hurdle is that many physicians, who now understand that social determinants of health are important, do not see addressing them as their responsibility. Patient movement from provider to provider and insurer to insurer also adds to the challenge of implementing a lifelong health and well-being approach.

ENGAGING HEALTH SYSTEMS IN IMPROVING POPULATION HEALTH

Magnan asked Knickman to discuss a recent diagram he developed of the key drivers of hospital investment in community health.[1] To support the efforts of the Robert Wood Johnson Foundation (RWJF) in promoting community health, Knickman and colleagues launched the Enhancing the Role of Hospitals in Improving Population Health (EHPH) Learning Center at NYU. Learning from the RWJF grantees, EHPH developed a framework of five main drivers of health system engagement in community and population health. Knickman briefly listed the drivers:

- **Health system mission or leadership that is focused on community health.** If leadership at the top is not engaged, "it's not going to happen," he said.
- **A business case.** Health systems need to have a reason to engage in population health, Knickman said. Reasons could include a return on investment, or relationship building and reputation as a community leader, for example.
- **Market concentration and competition.** Competitor health systems that contribute to community health improvements might attract staff and patients.

---

[1] See https://med.nyu.edu/chids/projects/enhancing-role-hospitals-improving-public-health (accessed June 23, 2021).

- **Multisector partnerships.** Transforming community health requires collaboration among health systems, community-based organizations, and other stakeholders.
- **Public policy and legislation.** Policies that require or incentivize investments in addressing the social determinants of health.

ALIGNING DRIVERS OF ACCOUNTABILITY AND ECONOMIC INTEREST

Magnan asked Pham to elaborate on the prospects of reaching a place where economic interests are aligned in a way that providers will be interested in population health and well-being. Pham said population health is a shared problem and providers cannot address it alone. The allocation of both accountability and resources for solving these issues is complex and involves multiple stakeholders. She said it is important to frame population health issues in terms that do not alienate stakeholders, and to facilitate "collective problem solving with everyone contributing proportionate to their means and their interests." A top-down approach would likely not be constructive, she said.

Pham applied several key economic concepts to suggest an approach for moving forward. First, top-down government intervention is not necessarily needed to solve big problems. There is a role for government, she continued, but government does not need to drive the conversations. Rather, the conversation can be organized by a trusted party in the community "that has credibility with multiple stakeholders, in multiple sectors, who have an interest in solving this problem." This could be a research institution, a philanthropy, or a convening organization that can bring stakeholders together.

Next, the trusted entity can gather input from stakeholders in a blinded fashion regarding what they might be willing and able to contribute to a solution. Pham noted that a blinded approach helps to reduce reputational posturing by stakeholders (i.e., stakeholders might not be realistic about what they can deliver and might overpromise in an unblinded setting). With a proposed collective pool of resources, the trusted entity can then begin to negotiate a solution without stakeholders feeling coerced. This approach, she said, results in a conversation about how to best use a unified pool of resources for collective action.

Knickman added that many individuals in the business community are adopting a double bottom-line approach that measures profits and return to investors, as well as social impact.

TAKING ACTION IN HEALTH CARE

Panelists discussed areas where leaders can work to facilitate the shift toward new values and investment priorities in health care. Pham emphasized the need to continue to make health care more efficient. She suggested that embracing a value-based path for the long term could ultimately allow organizations the freedom to invest creatively for health outcomes, rather than simply focusing on revenue-generating services.

Beyond efficiency, Pham suggested that a "fundamental contribution that providers can make is collecting the data." Data are needed on the current social circumstances and needs of patients, especially qualitative data on interactions and causal pathways that contribute to overall health and health care, she said. She emphasized that without these data, prioritizing investments is very difficult.

Knickman noted two key challenges: increasing investments in addressing the social determinants of health upstream, and identifying the drivers of community health and community development. He suggested that increasing the adoption of value-based payment would increase social- and community-based services. Developing the evidence base on which social services are most effective is also important.

Knickman also drew attention to the need to focus on and provide incentives for improving care for the most vulnerable, including those with complex chronic conditions, mental health and substance use conditions, and intellectual and developmental disabilities.

Another challenge, Knickman said, is how to implement "passive interventions that lead people to the right choices" and foster healthier communities. He suggested that health systems should take the lead and even include this in their mission. He observed that, while there has been interest from health system leadership, much of the activity has been "token" and not at scale.

POLICY CHANGES TO CONSIDER

Magnan asked panelists to suggest one policy change, at any level (national, local, private, public, etc.), to explore. If one action is going to be taken, Pham said, it should be to redesign the physician fee schedule. Absolute prices for care are important, but she suggested that the relative prices in the fee schedule are the larger problem. Under current payment approaches used by Medicare and other payers, the profit margin for providers varies according to the service. Furthermore, Pham said that clinical services with great care value, such as taking the time to talk to the patient, generate the lowest profit margin. Office-based procedures such as electrocardiograms generate much higher margins. Profit margins drive both physician behavior and facility investments in infrastructure that supports income-generating procedures. As a result, certain medical specialties become much more attractive for providers than other specialties, and certain types of initiatives are much more attractive for health systems. Even though providers and health systems understand and appreciate the broader societal goals, they respond to these underlying signals perpetuated by the fee schedule.

A challenge on the community resource side, Knickman said, is that investments made by a health system now will pay off over time, and people move from health system to health system during that time. He suggested addressing this concern by pooling resources for longer term investments in community health, drawing funding from health systems, payers, and others. Pham suggested that local government and local philanthropy contribute to the shared cost as well. She referred participants to the Vickrey-Clarke-Groves model of collective action and collective resource pooling.

DISCUSSION

Leadership for Change

Recalling the comments by Pham about reforming the physician fee schedule, Cathy Baase asked who could provide appropriate leadership for such policy changes. Pham responded that the leadership needed to address these large problems will come from multiple sources. She suggested that the Centers for Medicare & Medicaid Services and Congress would be ideally suited to lead physician payment reform, but that large payers also have an opportunity to lead in this area. She reiterated that the community can lead the solution process by pooling resources and negotiating consensus on solutions. Solutions need not be driven by government.

Knickman noted that the tradeoff between consolidation and competition is an ongoing debate in health economics. One solution to address the problems with the physician fee schedule, he said, would be "corporate medicine" (i.e., physicians work on salary for large health corporations). Similarly, having a limited number of health systems nationally would also solve some of the fee issues. Pham and Knickman both pointed out, however, that such an approach would require administered prices.

Market Forces

David Kindig of the University of Wisconsin–Madison mentioned a few examples of the progress made toward redirecting resources from the health care sphere toward health and well-being (e.g., ACOs, CMMI initiatives, shared savings). However, health care remains primarily fee-for-service. He observed that the market forces behind genomics, for example, have led to investment and infrastructure. He said definitions of value need to include population health and, in that regard, suggested there is a need to strengthen sectors such as early childhood education.

Pham agreed that the market forces behind genomics dwarf those behind early childhood education. She suggested that the current health care system would seem to be what people want. Despite assertions that everyone values community health and wants community well-being, people also still want access to top-level providers and coverage of expensive treatments that might only provide incremental value to the patient. "We want the long-term strategies, but we are seduced by new large buildings and new gadgets," she said. A national conversation is needed to define what people are willing to forgo to be able to fund community well-being.

Knickman commented that the current health system might be the right system for those who can afford it. However, it is not the right health system to meet the needs of the most vulnerable. He referred to the work of the Latino Community Foundation in California, which feels that meeting the health and education needs of the state's large Latino population is essential for the state's future economic prosperity.

Establishing the Evidence Base

Robert Kaplan of Stanford University continued on the topic of what will attract investors. For example, the idea that investments in genomic- or molecular biology–based interventions can lead to better health seems fairly widely accepted. The value of addressing the social determinants of health, however, is not clear to most people. From a provider perspective, there are established, evidence-based guidelines for managing cholesterol and blood pressure from the American Heart Association and the American College of Cardiology, Kaplan said, but there are no comparable guidelines for managing the social determinants of health. He asked about the status of building the evidence base to make the case for investing in behavioral and social determinants of health.

Magnan observed that data on social determinants of health are being collected, but what should be done with those data is not clear. Knickman emphasized the need for robust and integrated data systems and the ability to rapidly evaluate the data. He noted that relevant data can be found in electronic health record systems, claims systems, and other sources. Knickman shared an example from his laboratory of merging datasets to analyze how lowering speed limits in neighborhoods would impact accidents and pedestrian deaths. Pham suggested that the National Institutes of Health or the Agency for Healthcare Research and Quality could conduct a study akin to the National Health and Nutrition Examination Survey, but focused on understanding social factors and health. This could help to establish the dataset and research platform on which interventional studies could then be done.

Advocating for Health

Terry Allan of Ohio's Cuyahoga County Board of Health recalled comments made by the panelists about the value of a collective and collaborative approach to reinvestment. He shared an example regarding efforts to reduce racial disparities in infant mortality in the Greater Cleveland area that he said involved "unprecedented collaboration among medicine, public health, government, and payers." Another example is the support for comprehensive smoke-free laws in Ohio, which he said is the result of a lot of advocacy work. Allen observed that, while a collaboration might be successful, it can often be short lived as collaborators must return to their usual responsibilities. He suggested that advocacy from the medical community could influence elected officials with regard to payment and spending priorities in ways that health-related collaborations and initiatives could have more lasting impact.

Knickman agreed with the importance of advocacy. He noted that there are many networks advocating in "relentless, quiet ways," engaging chief executive officers and chief financial officers to ensure they understand why community health and well-being is so important. He observed that advocacy by health systems can sometimes create tension with community-based health organizations that might feel threatened by large academic health systems. He added that advocacy efforts, whether at the grassroots level or by organizations, need more funding.

Pham said it is generally agreed that efforts should focus on those who have the greatest need and who are underserved. However, she added that the uncomfortable reality of the marketplace is that it is easier to get the attention of investors by focusing on the populations they prize economically. She pondered what might happen if there were consumer demand by Medicare beneficiaries, consumers with private insurance, or their advocates for more attention to addressing the social determinants of health. How might providers alter their behavior to meet the expectations of consumers they value economically? How might that behavior then naturally extend to benefit needier and less profitable populations? Pham observed that younger patients prefer convenience when getting clinical care and prefer providers who acknowledge the circumstances of their work and lives. They are "far less interested in ... fancy facilities," she said, and suggested this could be leveraged to draw the attention of the market toward the community.

4

Evolving Values and Priorities Among Business Investors

The second panel discussed why and how values and priorities are changing in the capital markets, and how investors who supply funds and those who use investment capital interact. Maurice Jones of Local Initiatives Support Corporation (LISC), an organization that uses capital to support community revitalization projects, provided perspective from the demand side of the relationship. Lisa Williams of Goldman Sachs shared her perspective from the capital supply side. The session was moderated by Lisa Richter of Avivar Capital. (Highlights of this session are presented in Box 4-1.)

USING CAPITAL TO DRIVE CHANGE

In 1968, the Ford Foundation originated the use of "program-related investments" for charitable purposes, Richter said, because it believed that grants they had made to organizations in low-income communities were not leading to improved conditions in those communities. She suggested this was one of the first examples of values beginning to change among business investors in the United States. The idea was to provide investment capital (through loans) that would allow organizations in low-income communities to participate in the capital markets. Around the same time, Richter continued, groups of religious women were also using their resources to invest in their communities. Nuns invested in both grassroots lending efforts and voted their shares to push corporations to divest from South Africa and support the dismantling of apartheid.

> **BOX 4-1**
> **Key Points Made by Individual Speakers***
>
> - Sustainable and responsible impact investing has expanded beyond community development to encompass investments that can drive improvements in population health. (Richter)
> - Community development financial institutions (CDFIs) work on the demand side, leveraging capital to drive change in underserved communities. (Richter)
> - The role of Local Initiatives Support Corporation (a CDFI) is to be the first capital investor in a disinvested community, taking a first loss position so that more traditional financial institutions will follow and stack capital to drive change at the scale needed. (Jones)
> - For a range of reasons (e.g., infrastructure, technical capacity, incentives), community development is more challenging in rural areas than urban areas. (Jones)
> - Access to capital is itself a health determinant. (Richter)
> - Incorporating community voice into investment decisions is important. (Williams)
>
> ---
>
> * This list is the rapporteur's summary of the main points made by individual speakers and participants (noted in parentheses) and does not reflect any consensus among workshop participants, or endorsement by the National Academies of Sciences, Engineering, and Medicine.

People were starting to look at where money was going and the impact of those investment choices on communities.

Five decades later, the fields of impact investing, socially responsible investing, or most recently, sustainable and responsible impact investing, have expanded beyond community development to encompass environmental preservation, asset building, education, and the application of technology across education, health, finance, and other sectors. Over the past decade attention has been paid to how these investment tools can be applied to drive improvements in population health, Richter added. In addition, community development financial institutions (CDFIs) have been created to leverage capital to drive change in underserved communities. One example of a CDFI is LISC.

DEMAND SIDE PERSPECTIVE: LOCAL INITIATIVES SUPPORT CORPORATION

LISC was established 40 years ago as one of the first recipients of a program-related investment from the Ford Foundation, Jones said. Like others in the field at the time, the initial focus of LISC was to provide local neighborhood-based community development corporations with access to capital so they could revitalize abandoned real estate and "catalyze a market for housing in those neighborhoods." In the 1990s, he continued, LISC recognized that addressing housing was not sufficient to revitalize neighborhoods. LISC evolved beyond housing to invest in broader aspects of community development such as financing small businesses, entrepreneurs, schools, and community facilities. The role of LISC, Jones explained, is to be the first capital investor in a disinvested community, taking a first loss position so that more traditional financial institutions will follow and stack capital (e.g., philanthropic, corporate, government). To date, LISC has invested $20 billion in disinvested communities, which has leveraged an additional $60 billion from other investors. Richter expanded on the concepts of first loss position and capital stack. This means, she said, that LISC is willing to bear more risk (i.e., take more of the potential losses) than the follow-on lenders. By providing this type of credit enhancement or risk mitigation, LISC can attract significant investor capital from other lenders, which, stacked together, can help to drive change at the scale needed.

Community Development in Rural Versus Urban Communities

Richter asked Jones to comment on the differences between rural communities and urban communities with regard to community development. A key difference, Jones said, is that it can be more difficult to attract investment capital for rural communities due to the relatively low population density. Another difference is that there is generally less infrastructure and less technical capacity among neighborhood-based groups in most of rural America to support the project work and produce results. In addition, there are often fewer incentives to attract capital to rural areas. As an example, Jones mentioned the Community Reinvestment Act, which requires banks to extend credit to help those in the communities in which they do business. Jones noted that this currently means localities where banks have a physical presence, and many low-income areas are devoid of bank branch offices. Lastly, he suggested that government capacity to handle sophisticated financial transactions is generally weaker in rural areas than urban areas.

Jones emphasized that even though community development is more challenging in rural areas than urban areas, it is still being done. LISC works in 2,000 rural counties in 44 states and has a $450 million outstanding loan portfolio. Another challenge, Richter said, is that many communities, both urban and rural, do not have a local CDFI like LISC.

Connecting Community Development and Health

Richter reiterated that increasing attention has been paid over the past decade to the association between health and community development. She referred to the data discussed by Adams (see Chapter 2) and the county health rankings developed by Kindig and colleagues,[1] which indicate that at least 70 percent of population health outcomes can be traced to community factors (e.g., the built environment, socioeconomic factors, access to and quality of care). "If we don't build communities where people can make healthy choices," Richter said, "we can't expect to realize that vision of population health." She suggested that this acknowledgment of the association between health and community development gave new meaning to the work of LISC and other CDFIs, and she asked if it impacted LISC's strategy or approach to measuring impact.

LISC recently announced that it would invest $10 billion over 10 years in underinvested and disinvested communities, Jones said. These new investments will be directed toward improving health metrics. Since its inception, he said, LISC has partnered with financial institutions, but moving forward, the values and mission of LISC are more strongly aligned with the health sector. LISC has hired staff for a health care team and will work closely with health care partners. The first partner is ProMedica in Toledo, Ohio. Jones said a $45 million social determinants of health fund has been established that will be used over 7 to 10 years to address social determinants of health in uptown Toledo, including housing, economic development, and workforce development. ProMedica had observed disproportionate use of emergency department services for conditions related to social determinants of health by residents from this area. Jones noted that, in general, there can be a 10- to 30-year difference in life expectancy between low-income Census tracts and more affluent Census tracts. Metrics assessed will include the numbers of housing units revitalized and jobs created, as well as hospital readmission rates and metrics that can inform ProMedica's operations. Similar partnerships are now being established with other hospitals. Jones said the hospitals have an understanding of the health and wellness needs of the residents, and LISC has the established relationships with community-based partners that are essential to progress of the initiatives. He emphasized the importance of building relationships and trust and taking the time to understand the needs and aspirations of the partner health care organizations.

In summary, Richter said, LISC functions on the demand side, working to raise capital and redeploy it to address social determinants of

---

[1] For more information, see https://pophealth.wisc.edu/news/population-health-institute-measures-us-health-county-health-rankings-roadmaps (accessed June 23, 2021) and http://www.countyhealthrankings.org (accessed June 23, 2021).

health. In this regard, she said, "access to capital is itself a health determinant." The flow of capital is often unseen, and therefore is not often thought considered. However, the effects of capital investment can be powerful, and she said the partnerships being created by LISC have the potential to amplify the effects of capital investments for health.

SUPPLY SIDE PERSPECTIVE: GOLDMAN SACHS

Lisa Williams of Goldman Sachs shared insights from the work of helping institutions in aligning their capital with their values. Two considerations include the nature of the organization and its intent. The clients for impact investing services range from high net worth individuals to institutional offices, and they work toward a spectrum of impact and returns. Some clients, such as family offices, have a geographic focus in maximizing their returns, Williams noted. Interest areas for others may include environmental and social goals, and for some institutions, their stakeholders want to know that the capital that finances businesses or other investments is aligned with the population being served. Williams offered pension pools as an example, adding that if they are for food industry workers, the investors would seek alignment with the employees' work. The perspective in shaping the entire assets of an institution goes beyond the philanthropic, and includes attention to asset allocation (e.g., bonds, stocks, private venture), Williams noted. If the goal is a more healthy and equitable community, what might investments look like?

Williams said on the public market side,[2] investment proximity to impact may be most important. Investors may not want exposure to tobacco or fossil fuels, and the high-level themes for investing will be health and well-being, for example, in companies that are transitioning to value-based care. On the private market side, there are growing investments in traditional companies that are creating innovations around health. For example, Williams said, administrative burden and poor coordination of care lead to waste, so investors look at businesses that transform how health care is done. That could include companies looking to automate "low-value" tasks to enable more clinician time with patients. In the domain of affordable housing, the opportunities are found in looking at specific populations in need of affordable housing, such as people with intellectual disabilities, and "asking how to create safe, quality housing and do that in an institutional way, and working with hospitals to facilitate this."

---

[2] That is, publicly traded as opposed to privately held companies.

Measuring Impact and Progress

During the discussion period, Williams responded to a question about quantifying impact by noting that qualitative examples and progress are needed because investors tend not to allocate capital by providing metrics to report on, but rather "ask what are key pieces that tie to the business" and how do they increase revenue, and how can progress be measured? Another important step, she added, is to communicate with people making the investment decisions, and to incorporate community voice wherever possible, perhaps through grant makers.

Cathy Baase asked whether the focus is on upstream versus downstream investments in health. Williams responded that some investors are interested in specific diseases, but some focus on technology to improve information sharing, logistics, and care. Richter added that there are health sector funders who are looking at upstream opportunities from housing to small business, who have a people–place–planet focus, who recognize that climate risk is human health risk, and who acknowledge that sectors such as education have a high impact on health later in life, therefore underscoring the importance of investing early in the life course or early in the disease course.

Jones commented that LISC partners with investors are helping to develop supermarkets, and engaging in efforts to develop housing, supermarkets, and financing for federally qualified health centers.[3] Paula Lantz of the University of Michigan commented on several years of research on pay-for-success financing—private and third (i.e., philanthropic) sector capital is raised and government pays it back if metrics for success are met—to address population health and social determinants of health issues. Lantz remarked that the model has promise and has had some success, but her research has also highlighted pitfalls. Jones responded that the private sector needs the bridge financing that pay-for-success models offer. In her response, Williams noted that fundamentals of a project could change over a few years, as stockholders and relationships evolve over the life of a bond—these are "very bespoke projects and hard to put into an easy Excel model." However, Williams added, pay-for-success financing is an important instrument and public–private partnerships are needed to maximize its potential.

Abhishek Pandey of New York University Langone Health asked how investors handle the long time needed to get answers to some questions or to observe outcomes of interventions. Williams answered that there

---

[3] For example, LISC partners with Morgan Stanley and The Kresge Foundation in the $200 million Healthy Futures Fund, which finances the development of federally qualified health centers. See http://www.lisc.org/our-initiatives/health/healthy-futures-fund (accessed June 23, 2021).

are constructs to help address that, such as fund lives that are 10 years or longer, including evolving evergreen funds, requiring people to be comfortable with their capital being locked up for a longer time line, and have a longer time horizon. What is needed in those cases, added Williams, are midterm metrics and other innovative structures to help mitigate the uncertainty associated with long time lines. Jones noted that it is hard to invest in early childhood because we do not know outcomes for 10, 20, even 30 years. Foundations can use program-related investment dollars to model successful interventions that can be scaled. Jones shared the example of LISC's $15 million fund for affordable housing, which includes among investors philanthropy, for-profit entities, and hospitals. Although the affordable housing issue probably will not be fixed in 15 to 20 years, progress can be made. Jones called this "patient" capital, adding that demanders of capital have the opportunity to orient or familiarize those supplying it with the idea that needs to be done over the long term, and thus help bring in new investors.

Mary Pittman of the Public Health Institute asked how investors deal with gentrification that displaces people who have lived in a community for a long time. Jones answered that anti-displacement tools are available, such as the creation of a housing fund in the Bay Area. The key, he added, is to implement investment and anti-displacement measures simultaneously.

5

Case Example of Investment by a Health Care Organization

Leaders from University Hospitals (UH) in Cleveland, Ohio, were invited to share their example of investment by a health care–sector organization. Patricia DePompei of UH Rainbow Babies & Children's Hospital and UH MacDonald Women's Hospital shared her perspective from the clinical side. Heidi Gartland, also of UH, provided a community engagement perspective on how UH became an anchor institution in the community. The panel was moderated by Gary Gunderson of Wake Forest Baptist Health and Stakeholder Health. Gunderson emphasized that this discussion is about "real neighborhoods," and about a health care leader sustaining their commitment to the real communities where their patients and employees live. (Highlights of this session are presented in Box 5-1.)

UH: STRIVING TOWARD A CULTURE OF POPULATION HEALTH

UH was founded in the Greater University Circle area of Cleveland in 1866. The UH system currently includes 18 hospitals and 40 health centers, and serves 1 million unique patients annually. The Greater University Circle area has experienced disinvestment over the years, Gartland said, and residents have experienced structural racism such as redlining (discriminatory lending practices based on the race and/or ethnicity of a neighborhood). The median household income in the Greater University Circle is $18,500, and one in two children live in poverty. Infant mortality is high (18.6 per 1,000 births) and disproportionately affects African American infants. The number of children under age 6 years with lead poisoning

> **BOX 5-1**
> **Key Points Made by Individual Speakers***
>
> - The University Hospitals (UH) anchor institution investment strategy is to "hire local, buy local, live local" and includes a focus on place-based community health and wellness. (Gartland)
> - UH revised its community health needs assessment from a primarily quantitative assessment to a more qualitative assessment that engaged the community. In response to the findings, UH convened a Community Advisory Board. (DePompei)
> - To meet the health care and community-based needs identified by the Community Advisory Board and patient/caregiver and provider surveys, UH opened the Rainbow Center for Women & Children as a new medical home in the community. (DePompei)
> - Creative initiatives need to be mission aligned and have a clear business case to garner leadership and stakeholder support and funding. Construction of the new center was fully funded through New Markets Tax Credits and philanthropy. (DePompei)
> - Lack of coordination across contractual arrangements with managed care organizations is a barrier to implementing a model of care for an entire population. (Gartland)
>
> ---
>
> * This list is the rapporteur's summary of the main points made by individual speakers and participants (noted in parentheses) and does not reflect any consensus among workshop participants, or endorsement by the National Academies of Sciences, Engineering, and Medicine.

is four times the national average. The unemployment rate is 24 percent, and many of those who need work have barriers to employment.

About 10 years ago, Gartland said, UH undertook an initiative to reinvest in the UH organization. As part of the planning process, it was decided that UH would not simply invest in its own infrastructure, but would also invest in its community to build health and wealth.

The Anchor Mission: Hire Local, Buy Local, Live Local

Initial thoughts, Gartland said, were that this initiative would be a one-time investment to build up the community, and then UH would step back. Instead, she continued, UH has established itself as an anchor institution, and investing in and interacting with the Greater University Circle area has "become a way of life." For details, Gartland referred participants to the report *The Anchor Mission: Leveraging the Power of Anchor Institutions to Build Community Wealth*, which analyzes the UH initiative as a case example of community investment.[1] Briefly, UH planned to invest $750 million in the local economy through a strategy of "hire local, buy local, live local."

Hire Local

The first element of this anchor strategy was to put an emphasis on hiring people from the local neighborhoods, especially those who were under- and unemployed. In partnership with community organizations, UH identified local residents who were interested in working in entry-level jobs at UH. Interested residents were provided with skills training, resume building, and interview training. Gartland said more than 1,000 people from the local community have been hired over the past 5 years for entry-level jobs. To make more entry-level jobs available, existing employees were also given opportunities to advance. In addition, several staffing programs were launched, including Step Up to UH, designed to develop a pipeline of incoming staff from the local community, and New Bridge, which trains people for jobs as phlebotomists, pharmacy technicians, nurses' aides, and other in-demand roles.

Buy Local

UH planned to put money into the local economy through engagement with local businesses, especially women-owned and minority-owned businesses. One example described by Gartland was a $1 million investment in the development of the Green City Growers neighborhood cooperative, from which UH could then purchase fresh produce. She noted that thus far, UH has purchased $300,000 worth of lettuce. A similar venture is a laundry cooperative, which now handles a portion of UH's massive laundry service needs. Gartland pointed out that many of the employees of these cooperatives are re-entry workers, local residents who have been incarcerated and have difficulty getting hired for good-paying jobs.

Live Local

UH encourages its employees to live locally by providing employees with financial and other assistance to help them purchase property, upgrade their existing homes, or rent in the surrounding communities. Gartland said several hundred employees have taken advantage of this program.

---

[1] Available at https://democracycollaborative.org/content/anchor-mission-leveraging-power-anchor-institutions-build-community-wealth (accessed June 23, 2021).

Health Local

UH has also embraced place-based community health and wellness as part of its anchor mission. Gartland noted the importance of the support of the UH leadership, including the Board and chief executive officer, which allowed them to take a different approach to investing than UH had done in the past. Together with the local county Board of Health, UH has been investing in equity and health in the local community.

Community Health Needs Assessment

DePompei elaborated on the UH investment in place-based community health and wellness—specifically, their efforts to address the health care needs of infants, children, and women in the communities that are direct neighbors of UH.

In 2015, UH updated its approach to its community health needs assessment, evolving from a primarily quantitative assessment to a more qualitative assessment that engaged the community. The response from the community was "loud and clear," DePompei said. The assessment found there was a lack of trust between the community and UH. There were aspects of health care that the community believed were not being sufficiently addressed, especially access to behavioral and mental health services and access to dental care. The assessment also revealed the need for UH to better engage the entire family, especially men, and pay more attention to multigenerational care.

In response to the findings of the community health needs assessment, in March 2016, UH convened a Community Advisory Board. Invitations were sent to patients and stakeholders from the community across a broad range of sectors. DePompei noted that there was 100 percent attendance by the invitees to the initial Community Advisory Board meeting, which she added was during an ice storm in sub-zero temperatures. This Community Advisory Board continues to have a very high level of participation and engagement, she continued.

Advice from the Community Advisory Board was to redesign the delivery of primary care for the women and children in the neighborhoods surrounding UH. DePompei said clinic services were housed on the first floor of Rainbow Babies & Children's Hospital, and these clinics were the main training sites for pediatric and obstetric/gynecologic residents. To understand the needs of patients and their families who are served by the Rainbow ambulatory pediatric practice and the MacDonald Women's and Children's obstetrics/gynecology service, a longitudinal patient/caregiver survey was conducted.

The survey response rate was high (80 percent). Patients and families reported significant health-related needs, and stress resulting from unmet needs. Social factors reported included housing instability, financial concerns and inability to pay bills, food insecurity, and transportation issues. DePompei noted that, even though about 85 percent of the families surveyed are employed, they often have low-paying jobs. Food insecurity was compounded by the lack of a local supermarket in the neighborhoods bordering UH. Lack of a direct bus line was a barrier to patient access to health care at the clinic.

Providers were also surveyed for input on what would be an ideal model of primary care delivery. Responding providers understood the need to address the social determinants of health, DePompei said, and they were interested in guidance on how to accomplish this while keeping up with busy clinic schedules.

A New Medical Home in the Community

In partnership with patients and families and the Community Advisory Board, UH set out to build a medical practice that would meet both health care and community-based needs. In July 2018, the Rainbow Center for Women & Children opened. DePompei noted that construction of the new center was fully funded through New Markets Tax Credits and philanthropy. The center, which she described as welcoming and vibrant, features artwork by local artists. Services include primary care pediatrics, obstetrics/gynecology, maternal–fetal medicine and imaging, dental, optometry, pharmacy, mental health and addiction services, a women/infants/children office, onsite legal aid, and social needs navigation. DePompei said that the center is so busy that additional bus stops and parking are being added.

Securing Funding and Internal Stakeholder Buy-In

Gunderson asked DePompei to elaborate on funding creative initiatives to meet community needs. The first point, she said, is that initiatives need to be part of the overall mission of the organization to garner support from leadership. For UH, the construction of the new center was clearly within its mission. One then needs a clear business case for the initiative, and this was more challenging, she said. Financially, 91 percent of the pediatric patients served by the clinic and 90 percent of the women are covered by Medicaid, which she said has generally poor reimbursement for primary care services. For that reason, it was important to rally support from community members by making them aware of the unacceptable community health statistics, such as the racial and geographic disparities in infant life expectancy in the surrounding neighborhoods versus nearby suburbs. Next, it was necessary to secure the funding for the capital project. DePompei said UH was encouraged by the Robert Wood Johnson Foundation to pursue New Markets Tax Credits. As noted earlier, the center was fully funded through New Markets Tax Credits and philanthropy. She added that the Ohio Department of Medicaid has funded many of the programs. As an example, she mentioned Centering Pregnancy, a group model of care delivery with proven results (e.g., reduced rates of preterm delivery). DePompei said they continue to look for ways to increase efficiency and drive more volume at the center to ensure sustainability.

New Markets Tax Credits are intended to incentivize development in economically distressed areas, and Gartland said the Greater University Circle area is one of the most economically underresourced areas in Northeast Ohio. She acknowledged the leadership and support from the Board for allowing the necessary legal structures to be implemented to secure the New Markets Tax Credits. This was a calculated risk for UH, Gartland said, but she explained that DePompei has a history of being able to deliver on projects and promises and had the trust of the Board to lead this effort. Gartland also noted that the local community development financial institutions were eager to participate in the development of the center. DePompei agreed and emphasized the value of New Markets Tax Credits "as a catalyst for economic growth." The intent is that the building of the anchor institution (in this case, the primary care center) will lead to other community growth, and she mentioned the opening of a grocery store and coffee shop in what had been a food desert.

Gunderson emphasized the point by Gartland about delivering on promises made to internal stakeholders and the community. He suggested that leaders who fulfill their promises create momentum and inspire others to partner in the initiatives. DePompei agreed and said that delivering on the promises made to patients and their families is the primary goal. As an executive, she must also ensure that regulatory requirements are met, and that profits and losses meet expectations.

Gartland called the process "a journey" that began with the UH Vision 2010 strategic plan that recognized the need to invest in the community. She mentioned that one of the earlier steps in the journey was a $12 million Center for Medicare & Medicaid Innovation (CMMI) Health Care Innovation Award in 2012. Part of the project included the building of a new office that was first slated for the suburbs, near where the providers lived, but was ultimately built in one of the Greater University Circle neighborhoods near UH, where the population to be served lived. Gartland noted the challenge of changing the mindset of the providers to begin to understand the importance of location. Later, having this office already in the Greater University Circle area helped with provider acceptance and support of locating the new center there as well.

Gunderson asked how young professionals entering the health care field are responding to these initiatives. An unexpected benefit of the new center, DePompei said, has been as a recruitment tool for top medical residents and other practitioners. Many up-and-coming residents, physicians, nurse practitioners, nurse midwives, and other practitioners understand the importance of addressing the social determinants and are excited by the work of the center.

DISCUSSION

Coordination Across Payers Serving a Population

Sanne Magnan asked the panelists to discuss the policy or system change they would most like to see made by their largest payer, Medicaid. Gartland said she would like to have much more coordination across contractual arrangements with managed care organizations. She noted the challenge of translating innovative total cost of care models across five separate contracts. Some payers are "more enlightened" with respect to population health, and others are less so, she said, which can be a barrier to implementing a model of care for an entire population. She suggested finding ways to incentivize payers to be more aligned with the care models that are reducing costs. Gartland also called for a share of the savings to be returned to the health system. DePompei concurred and said the state has supported the Centering Pregnancy Program because of the demonstrated cost savings from the reduction in neonatal intensive care unit admissions. There are many examples of how upstream interventions can reduce overall costs of care, but she added that the models must be sustainable. Magnan referred participants to a recent publication by Pham and Ginsburg on coordinating contracting in payment reform (Pham and Ginsburg, 2018).

Gauging Success

Alexander Rossides of Social Impact Exchange inquired about the size of the population being served by the center; whether the patient volume or revenue have increased sufficiently to confirm the economic argument for building the center; the population health outcomes and timeframes the center hopes to achieve; and the "gravitational pull" of the center in attracting other businesses to invest in the area.

Gartland said Cuyahoga County has a population of about 1 million, the city of Cleveland has a population of nearly 400,000, and the Greater University Circle area has just under 200,000. Demographically, she said, the East side is primarily African American and the West side is mostly white and Hispanic.

As an example of how UH has been a catalyst, she said that UH partnered with the county and city Boards of Health on developing a joint community health needs assessment in 2018, 2 years before a state requirement for joint needs assessments goes into effect in 2020. This has prompted other health systems to step up as well. She said that although health systems compete on patient care, there should not be competition on community health. From an economic perspective, Gartland said that UH has established itself as an anchor health care institution that continues to invest in the community, and other businesses are eager to be "anywhere UH is."

DePompei said that basic short- and longer-term health care delivery metrics were established as part of the original CMMI award (e.g., reducing emergency pediatric psychiatry inpatient admissions by addressing behavioral and mental health in outpatient visits; reducing the rate of children needing dental surgery due to untreated dental caries by applying fluoride varnish to newly erupted molars; increasing immunization rates). Other metrics being tracked include the no-show rate for patients at the pediatric and women's health clinics. She suggested that ease of access and respect for the patients have contributed to increased numbers of patients keeping appointments. From a growth perspective, the center was expected to have 45,000 patient visits annually, and a metric of 5 percent growth in patient volume was factored into the New Markets Tax Credit agreement. She expressed optimism and said that "the initial indicators are incredibly promising."

Going to Scale

Marc Gourevitch observed that the UH board and leadership were mission driven in embracing the Greater University Circle anchor strategy. He asked how boards and chief executive officers of other organizations that are less mission driven might be convinced to embrace "doing well by doing good." Gartland said the UH system has hospitals in other low-income, underserved neighborhoods and is working strategically to implement similar place-based approaches in areas of need. UH is also participating with other hospitals and organizations to spread the anchor mission more broadly, including The Root Cause Coalition and the Healthcare Anchor Network. She acknowledged that leadership support is essential.

Job Training

John Auerbach asked whether the anchor strategy included job creation or job training opportunities for the community. DePompei pointed out that New Markets Tax Credits applicants must indicate the number of new jobs that will be created as part of the capital project. She reiterated that the hire-local aspect of the strategy was a core component of the UH commitment to the community, and it included hiring locally for both the construction of the center and the staffing of the completed center. The Step Up to UH Program was launched to help local residents gain entry-level jobs in health care and to access ongoing workforce training needed for career advancement. Gartland mentioned the Bridge to Your Future workforce development program in association with local community colleges that helps employees to develop the skills needed to pursue a certification or college degree. There are also job coaches who help employees navigate the life challenges that impact continued employment. This has reduced the turnover rate for new employees from the community from 80 percent to less than 20 percent, she said.

Equity as the Core of Advancing Population Health

Terry Allan, health commissioner for Cuyahoga County, where UH is based, said the mandate from the state of Ohio to begin conducting coordinated county-level health assessments across multiple systems presents opportunities as well as uncertainties and challenges. For example, he noted that a given health system can have a wide reach, beyond a specific county's borders. He acknowledged the role of UH in working through the challenges as assessments are conducted to meet regulatory requirements and to advance population health in the communities. He noted that it was exciting to see the conversations happening across multiple health systems, and the new priorities being discussed. He also acknowledged the role of workshop participants in these conversations and their authority to make decisions based on the discussions. He specifically recognized Danielle Price of UH for her focus on ensuring that health equity is part of the conversation, reinforcing the need to deploy resources to address the "compounding disadvantages that a subset of the population deals with in underresourced communities." As the hospitals in a county or a region work toward population health, equity should be the "guiding principle," he said.

Competition and Collaboration

Milstein asked how the implementation of the anchor institution strategy has affected competition or collaboration among UH and the other systems in the area. Those institutions include Case Western Reserve University and the Cleveland Clinic in the Greater University Circle area, and MetroHealth to the west. Gartland said she is chair of The Center for

Health Affairs, the local hospital association for Northeast Ohio. It serves as the convener for the collective community health needs assessments and as a place to work collaboratively. She mentioned several community health initiatives that the health systems have worked on collectively, for example, First Year Cleveland, which is focused on reducing infant mortality, and the Northeast Ohio Hospital Opioid Consortium. She noted that federal antitrust regulations prohibit the health systems from discussing the core business aspects of their care delivery, but allow the systems to work together to address issues of public health. She suggested that the anchor mission of hire local, buy local, live local is not competitive. Similarly, although UH might have been first to step into the community health space, all of the health systems are now working collaboratively. The chief executive officers of the health systems meet regularly, which she said was important for being servant leaders to the community. DePompei added that the health systems joke about "stealing shamelessly from each other," meaning that if one has shown success with a community health effort, such as the new UH center in the Greater University Circle area, the others should try to replicate it in their communities.

6

A Case Example of Business Investment

A leader from U.S. Trust at Bank of America Private Wealth Management was invited to share an example of business-sector investment with an orientation toward health and well-being. Jamie Rantanen of U.S. Trust at Bank of America shared his perspective as an institutional client advisor. The session was moderated by Catherine Baase of the Michigan Health Improvement Alliance and The Dow Chemical Company. (Highlights of this session are presented in Box 6-1.)

U.S. TRUST AT BANK OF AMERICA: IMPACT INVESTING

"Bank of America is one of the largest financial providers to the health care industry," Rantanen said, extending more than $35 billion in capital to the U.S. health care sector. U.S. Trust is the wealth management arm of Bank of America. Founded in the mid-1800s, U.S. Trust is the oldest and largest private bank in the United States and was acquired by Bank of America in 2007 to serve its ultra-high net worth investors. A specific team is dedicated to serving institutional nonprofit clients, endowments, and foundations. There is also a team of specialists who work with health care organizations both on aligning their mission and investment portfolio, and on organizational development (e.g., sustainability, impact measurement, donor development).

Bank of America developed its first environmental, social, and governance (ESG) manual in 2008, Rantanen continued. The ESG is the company's responsible growth strategy and stems from the lessons learned in the 2007–2008 financial crisis. It is updated annually and is now more

> **BOX 6-1**
> **Key Points Made by Individual Speakers***
>
> - Data on the environmental, social, and governance (ESG) activities of companies are now more readily available to investors, but many do not realize they can be intentional in their investments. (Rantanen)
> - Intangible assets contribute significantly to a company's value and "the best way to understand the values and risks of those assets is to use ESG data." (Rantanen)
> - Investment firms have an opportunity to guide investors in deploying significant capital into ESG-directed portfolios that are both high impact and high yield. (Rantanen)
> - In place-based impact investing, recognizing the difference between outputs and outcomes/impact is important. (Richter)
>
> _____
>
> * This list is the rapporteur's summary of the main points made by individual speakers and participants (noted in parentheses) and does not reflect any consensus among workshop participants, or endorsement by the National Academies of Sciences, Engineering, and Medicine.

than 100 pages, he said.[1] Rantanen noted that U.S. Trust has served some families for eight generations, and he observed that impact investing is of particular interest to the younger generations. The older generations are also taking notice of impact investing because of the strong interest of their heirs in ESG issues. By working with multigenerational clients, Rantanen said, firms like U.S. Trust have a "great opportunity to shepherd significant capital into very high-impact and well-run fiduciary portfolios for the future that are both doing well and good."

Investing in Health

Rantanen said each of the ESG categories—environmental, social, and governance—is grounded in health. When considering where to invest in health care in the public markets, Bank of America looks to companies engaged in healthy food, fitness, medical research and diagnostics, disease prevention, disease treatment, access to health care, employee benefits, agricultural technology, air quality, water quality, and product safety, for example. Bank of America chooses not to invest in companies that he said are "negatively impacting environmental and social-related

_____
[1] For the most recent ESG report, see https://about.bankofamerica.com/en/making-an-impact/esg-reports (accessed June 23, 2021).

health care issues." These would be companies that deal in unhealthy food, alcohol, tobacco, gambling, or adult entertainment, for example, or those that are toxic polluters or do not pay a living wage or provide standard employee benefits.

Baase asked whether those companies that Bank of America chooses not to invest in based on the company's portfolio or actions are aware they have been passed over, and why. "Impact investing and mission alignment investing are a growing force in the market," Rantanen said. Data on the ESG activities of companies have become more readily available to investors over the past decade. Still, he said, many investors do not realize that they can be intentional in their investments.

From the corporate perspective, many large companies are focused on ESG. First, Rantanen said, these companies embrace a fiduciary responsibility to "do no harm" and reduce their exposure to marketplace risks. Second, many seek to become known as a mission-driven brand (e.g., sustainable practices, healthy outcomes). Third, many companies are taking climate change into consideration in their actions (e.g., adopting sustainable agriculture practices to produce healthy food for an expanding population).

Socially Innovative Investing Platform

Socially Innovative Investing is a platform created by U.S. Trust for impact investing in the public markets. The platform, launched 6 years ago, incorporates ESG criteria and sustainable development goals when designing public market equity and bond portfolios. There are currently portfolios centered around low carbon, religious views and values, global equality, women and girls, and community health, and new portfolios are being developed. Over the past 5 years, most of these portfolios have outperformed the benchmarks, Rantanen said. Portfolio development starts with a financial analysis, but then takes into account ESG information that most investors are not considering. A recent quantitative equity strategy report on ESG by Merrill Lynch (another division of Bank of America) found that up to 68 percent of the value of S&P 500 companies is based on intangible assets, and Rantanen said that "the best way to understand the values and risks of those assets is to use ESG data."[2] Having established the financial and ESG analytics-based arguments for such thematic portfolios, investment firms can work with endowment, foundation, or individual investors to be more intentional and mission aligned in their investing.

---

[2] See https://about.bankofamerica.com/en/making-an-impact/esg-reports (accessed June 23, 2021).

Case Example

As a case example of impact investing in the public markets, Rantanen described how U.S. Trust and Avivar Capital helped a regional community foundation develop an investment portfolio around the theme of community health impact. The community health foundation sought to create a platform for local, place-based community health impact investments. Rantanen noted that these types of investment opportunities can be difficult to identify and access. A challenge was trying to use traditional public market asset classes to mission align their portfolio, and no existing platform had the right blend of broad perspective on health and environment with local, place-based investments for health. Together, U.S. Trust and Avivar Capital, a private place-based investment advisor, created a broad custom portfolio of national and international investments across asset classes that still maintained a community impact-driven focus on health.

The main lessons thus far, Rantanen said, are that community organizations are very focused on making community-level investments that can improve health locally, and that investing in the "bigger picture" can be aligned with this goal. For example, large national public companies are often the biggest employers in a community, and their actions can significantly affect employee and community health.

Expanding Focus on Impact Investing

Interest in impact investing is growing. Rantanen said many large investment firms have, like Bank of America, created platforms to support the increasing scale of impact-directed investments. He added that there are also many small organizations as well. "The impact investing ecosystem is very young," he said, but it has great potential. In addition, there is potential at the intersection of philanthropy and impact investing. He said that professional advisors, like himself, are being engaged to help develop impactful portfolios. He said investors, both individual and institutional, should challenge their current advisors to be attentive to ESG factors when recommending or making investments for them. He personally speculated that, in the coming 5 to 10 years, ESG due diligence would be a fiduciary requirement. He added that the Department of Labor now mandates that trustees of Employee Retirement Income Security Act plans assess ESG as part of their fiduciary responsibility.

DISCUSSION

Measuring Impact

Recalling Rantanen's comments on the expanding interest in impact investing and the increasing number of advisors and firms involved, Magnan asked him to comment on measures of success to determine whether these investments are impacting health, well-being, and equity over the next 5 to 10 years. Rantanen said "the revolution of ESG in portfolios" has peaked, and the focus for the coming decade is improving impact measurement and reporting of outcomes. Some firms that offer impact investments are already measuring and reporting outcomes. He suggested that impact measurement and transparent reporting of outcomes at the company level will be factored into a company's marketplace value. An "impact performance track record" could be used to de-risk investments, he said.

Mary Pittman asked about the types and sources of data that are used to inform impact investing, in particular, whether sources such as public health databases and information on hospital community benefits are being used to identify areas of need and potential investment. Rantanen said there are specialist advisors who "begin with the end in mind" and consider the outcomes desired and the measurements of success at the forefront when planning to invest. Lisa Richter of Avivar commented that they often work backward, first defining the outcome they hope to achieve, determining whether capital is needed to accomplish it, and how the end result will be measured. She noted that, in place-based impact investing, it is important to recognize the difference between outputs and outcomes/impact. For example, units of housing are an output, but the outcome indicator is who is living in the housing (e.g., have low-income residents been displaced/priced out?). Richter emphasized the value of partnerships, which can bring together complementary expertise, for example, bringing together community-level knowledge with the ability to bring initiatives to scale through investment initiatives.

ESG-Informed Investing in Practice

Bobby Milstein suggested that, over the coming decade, ESG could evolve to become routine institutional practice in investing. He asked about training the next generation of ESG advisors, and the incorporation of population health science. He suggested that a fuller understanding of the evidence needs could help to inform the research agenda and, correspondingly, the investment agenda. Rantanen said the U.S. Forum for Sustainable and Responsible Investment offers training to advisors in the market. The CFA Institute (which administers the Chartered Financial

Analyst program) now includes ESG in its required curriculum. Within organizations there is ESG training for interested portfolio managers, but he described it as "opt-in." However, he asserted, portfolio managers who do not adapt to the ESG movement over the coming decade are not likely to retain many clients. "Outcomes and the impacts are the next big chapter, and our platforms are going to just get better and better," he said. Bank of America is actively conducting due diligence to be able to expand the number of investment options on its impact platform. He added that due diligence process will need to evolve to be able to evaluate the risk and return of these impact investment products as they can be constructed differently.

Milstein also asked if working with multigenerational investors changes the investment strategy because there is the potential for a long-term outlook, and whether those families might be more directly engaged in the screening of potential investments. Rantanen responded that perhaps a long-term platform could be developed based on the family's interests, perhaps making angel/seed investments or providing venture capital to family-owned businesses that align the family's thematics.

Marc Gourevitch asked what proportion of investments are currently informed by ESG. Rantanen responded that it is easier to take ESG into account when investing in large companies in the public market because their track records are more available to compare. Trying to take ESG into account is more challenging when investing in small-cap stocks. A company's ESG information is also becoming easier to access in the private market.

7

Reflections on Leadership Investment Priorities

For the last agenda item, Phyllis Meadows of The Kresge Foundation facilitated a small group exercise that allowed participants to reflect on the day's discussions and apply lessons learned through role-playing as leaders in health care or business investment. To conclude the workshop, Joshua Sharfstein offered his closing comments and called on roundtable members and participants to share their final observations.

LEADERSHIP INVESTMENT: SMALL GROUP ACTIVITY

Workshop participants broke into four groups to consider investment priorities for health and well-being, as well as organizational and leadership challenges, for the fictional city of Ourlandia. The story of Ourlandia was introduced by Meadows, and a set of questions was provided to guide small group conversations. Group participants were invited to consider the scenario and questions from the perspective of a hypothetical hospital board in Ourlandia (i.e., a local health care leader) or the perspective of a pension fund manager (i.e., a business investment leader). A summary of the activity is provided in Box 7-1, with complete exercise materials provided in Appendix F.

> **BOX 7-1**
> **Investing for Value in Ourlandia**
>
> Ourlandia is a fictitious mid-size American city, once the nation's leading manufacturer of industrial glass. The city has seen many changes in recent years. Although it made its fortune in the glass industry, manufacturing has since declined, and city leaders have been slow in planning for socioeconomic transition. The population has declined by 15 percent over the past 30 years, and the expectation is that it will continue to fall. Ourlandia is a diverse community with a broad range of social challenges, including residential segregation. The community has extreme inequalities in wealth, poverty, and educational status. The health status of the community is also shifting. Residents suffer from chronic illnesses; rates of addiction and suicide are on the rise; and life expectancy has fallen. More than 60 percent of the residents believe the next generation of Ourlandians will be far worse off than their parents.
>
> Still, there are many civic assets. Ourlandians have inclusive values and a pioneering spirit. They are hardworking, pragmatic people who are willing to work across differences to respond to the emerging problems. There is trust in the community leaders. The health care and business sectors have invested in the community. The main hospital has become an anchor institution. Small companies and local banks have begun to invest in community development. A large pension fund is also embracing socially responsible investing.
>
> With this background in mind, consider the following (from the perspective of a health care leader or a business investment leader):
>
> 1. What are the most compelling priorities to enhance value for your organization and for Ourlandia?
> 2. How do these priorities reposition your role in Ourlandia?
> 3. What tradeoffs did you consider when setting your priorities?
> 4. What leadership challenges will you have to overcome in order to invest?
>
> SOURCE: Meadows presentation, December 3, 2018.

Leadership Investment Proposals: Small Group Reports[1]

Upon reconvening in plenary session, a rapporteur from each small group shared the outcome of the participants' discussion and their proposals for hypothetical leadership investments.

---

[1] This small group exercise was intended to engage participants in using what they had learned thus far in the workshop. This section of the proceedings summarizes the small group discussions based on the report by each group's designated rapporteur and should not be construed as reflecting any consensus of the group. All group responses and proposals reported are hypothetical and for only discussion purposes.

Hospital Board Group 1

Malcolm Fox of Culture of Health for Business reported for the first group, which approached the task from the perspective of a hospital board. Per the task, the board is seeking to reposition their nonprofit hospital as a high-value producer of health and well-being for all. Fox noted that there was somewhat of a split among the "board members." Some wanted to forge ahead with the repositioning initiative, while others believed there was a greater need to address the acute and chronic health issues within the community by focusing on the primary mission of being a provider of health care services. In other words, participants underscored an interest in investments that are attentive to both the short-term immediate health care needs and the longer-term growth initiatives for the hospital's future in the community.

Given $45 million per year for community health improvement, Fox reported that participants in the hypothetical hospital board decided to dedicate a portion of that funding to address some immediate health-related needs in the community, including infrastructure and housing. To identify the areas of immediate need, "board members" would engage key members of the business community, chamber of commerce, and the local government, Fox said. In addition, participants decided that a much broader community health needs assessment was needed for Ourlandia, and that expert stakeholder committees would be engaged to ensure high levels of community involvement. Another portion of the funding would then be put toward addressing the issues identified, for both immediate needs and long-term strategy investments.

Meg Gilmartin of the National Kidney Foundation added that the hypothetical board was diverse and included hospital staff (nurses, physicians), community members, housing advocates, community advocates, United Way, members of the business community including a local biotechnology firm, and a leading financial institution. She reported that participants identified the need for greater investment by the hospital in training, both for medical staff as well as for new growth (e.g., vocational training). Another suggestion was to invest in making transportation more accessible. Some participants emphasized the need to focus on areas that the hospital, as a health care organization, could uniquely address as a leader, and to also motivate the business community and the broader community to address other fundamental issues that are more outside of the health purview. The sense of hypothetical board members, she said, was that "keeping the status quo was not going to be sufficient."

In discussing what would be most critical to address, Fox reported that there were strong advocates on the board for housing, transportation, and child care for hospital staff. He noted the need to be transformative and invest for the future while still addressing the immediate needs of the community.

Pension Fund Group 1

Gary Gunderson reported for the first group that addressed the task from the perspective of pension fund managers. He noted that "the fundamental structures of public health and pension funds are radically different," which made it challenging for this group of public health professionals to role-play as pension fund managers. He said there are fundamental differences between how the $20 billion in assets would be managed from a public health perspective versus the perspective of a pension fund with a fiduciary obligation to retirees. There were also uncertainties in the parameters of the exercise that would impact investment recommendations the group would make. For example, knowing how many of the 200,000 covered members lived in Ourlandia would impact whether significant investments should be made to revitalize the local community where members lived, versus an obligation to members of the fund to maximize the return on investment of the $20 billion in assets. Another challenge noted was the 20-year time horizon of the exercise, which excludes funding some public health interventions known to have high returns on investment for the community over the longer term, such as early childhood education. Gunderson reported that group members also pondered how the pension might be structured in a way that encouraged potential recipients to stay in Ourlandia, or to postpone retirement if they were physically able.

Hospital Board Group 2

Mylynn Tufte, state health officer for North Dakota, summarized the discussions of the second group to consider investing from the perspective of a hospital board. The "board members" discussed the need for a more sustainable business model, she said, and considered the potential for "mergers to increase market share and purchasing power." Priorities identified by individual participants were "to be more of a team player," and "multisector accountability, owning the leadership role, and accepting diversity," she said. The hypothetical board said there had been protests outside during one of their meetings and they recognized that it was "something that we needed to be more accountable for," Tufte relayed. In considering safety, criminal justice reform, and public health, it was discussed that $1 billion of the endowment would be used to focus on education, workforce, and private-sector recruitment. The group also discussed possibly renaming the city, Tufte added.

Other participants acknowledged it would be challenging for leadership to secure buy-in for spending endowment funds on these priorities and initiatives. Another challenge would be catalyzing a culture shift, including helping to convey "how much short-term pain you are going to have to endure for this long-term gain," Tufte said. As one approach to building resilience and hope in the Ourlandia community, the board suggested commissioning a promotional video. Tufte shared as an example a video that was recently disseminated by the Fargo, North Dakota, police department promoting unity.[2]

Meadows commented that, even though the case scenario for the exercise focused on the negative aspects of Ourlandia and its recent decline, the community still has many admirable assets. She noted that "communities feel the weight of those negative figures and facts," and rebranding the city, including choosing a new name, can be an effective leadership strategy.

Pension Fund Group 2

Ivana Vaughn of The New York Academy of Medicine reported for the second group that addressed the task from the perspective of pension fund managers. In "doing well by doing good for Ourlandia," the pension fund managers prioritized developing an approach that would allow for both local investment in the community as well as national and international investments that would generate returns for Ourlandia. The underlying goal the managers sought to achieve was "lifelong economic security for families" through both financially and socially responsible investing. Some participants discussed creating a fund for local investments and seeking guidance from pension managers with environment, social, and governance (ESG) portfolio expertise, and using social impact bonds. Priorities for investment that were discussed included vocational technical education, early childhood education, safety, social and criminal justice, and natural resources protection. The pension fund managers also identified tourism as an important local resource and discussed increasing mass transit as well as hotel and conference space and entertainment venues. The managers would apply a health equity lens to all investments, Vaughn said.

In taking on these investment priorities, the hypothetical pension fund managers would be taking a much more active role in helping to revitalize Ourlandia. They would also be more accountable as community members by, for example, working to decrease waste and increase efficiency through their investment choices in the different sectors. Group participants recognized that transitioning from a traditionally passive role in the community to an active role would require some internal restructuring of the pension fund organization to ensure the short- and

---

[2] The "It's Time" video shown at the workshop can be viewed at https://www.youtube.com/watch?v=m53bk1Cta6A (accessed June 23, 2021).

long-term sustainability of the investments and to cover the increased administrative expenses. Participants also recognized that there was no guarantee that this new structure and approach to investing would be successful in achieving the desired goals.

Finally, Vaughn said, "fund managers" recognized that institutional leadership might need to address resistance, both internally and from the community and stakeholders, to this restructuring. Some participants noted the need to maintain trust between the leaders and the constituents and emphasized the importance of involving local residents in the conversation.

Discussion

Following the small group reports, Terry Allan expressed his appreciation for the exercise and said it is a plausible scenario that many communities today are facing. The industries in a community will vary, and the path forward will be different, but the need to reimagine their future is common across many communities.

Meadows asked whether the groups considered how their proposed solutions might address the growing inequalities in Ourlandia. Gunderson pointed out that many existing assets were accumulated over decades and under values and rules that are different from those being embraced today (e.g., a focus on equity). As politics and administrations change, it can be challenging to align those existing assets with new values and rules. He suggested that "the challenge is more fundamental than technical" and relates not to deciding where the fund should be invested, but to the fundamental structure, accountability, and rules that constrain the use of those funds. The challenge, he continued, is to influence changes to the rules. In that regard, Meadows observed that some of the groups proposed restructuring to become less passive and more active in the community. She pondered what leadership activities would be needed to make this type of shift in the face of existing governance structures and historical patterns of giving. Some highlights from the small group discussion are provided in Box 7-2.

A participant emphasized the importance of raising awareness of the association between health and the economy. She suggested that developing enduring economic health in a community like Ourlandia is more challenging than addressing social determinants of health such as housing or transportation in that community.

Another participant pointed out that the hypothetical hospital board assembled for the exercise might not represent how board discussions are held in many organizations. For example, a board might not engage the diverse range of community stakeholders in planning and decisions

> **BOX 7-2**
> **Highlights from Reporting Back on the Small Group Discussion***
>
> - Residents of a community are often not seen as assets because they are "under a dark cloud of economic and health challenges," and leadership is needed from individuals such as those participating in the workshop to maintain the momentum in addressing these issues in communities. (Meadows)
> - Governance discussions held by hospital boards may not resemble the hypothetical board discussions during the exercise, and fundamental shifts in governance thinking and approaches are likely required to change how boards operate and how they consider community views. (A participant)
> - Bold and out-of-the-box thinking may be more likely or easier to undertake during a crisis than during routine and positive conditions. (Gunderson)
> - An institution's board may need to manage tension between the need to be attentive to the short-term immediate health care needs of its patient population and the longer-term growth initiatives needed for the hospital's future in the community. (Fox)
>
> ---
>
> * This list is the rapporteur's summary of the main points made by individual speakers and participants (noted in parentheses) and does not reflect any consensus among workshop participants, or ondorsement by the National Academies of Sciences, Engineering, and Medicine.

that the hypothetical boards did. It would be a fundamental shift in governance conversations to change how the agenda is set and how the input from the community is used. It might also shift the decisions made in terms of "how big of a bet do you play versus protecting the long-term assets of the hospital," she said.

As an example of leadership changing the role of a hospital, Sanne Magnan shared how Lake Region Healthcare chief executive officer Larry Schulz was direct with his board about the need to engage the community and develop a rural health model for the future, underscoring a rural health, not a rural health care, model. She added that Schulz acknowledged that leaders would likely "hear things that we don't want to hear" from the community, but that a new direction was needed.

Meadows prompted participants to consider the similarities and differences among what the hospital board groups and the pension fund manager groups reported about their discussions. A participant observed that each group initially stayed within their defined roles and were perhaps constrained by those roles. When board members began to think beyond their traditional roles, there was more creativity in addressing the health and economic well-being of the community.

Meadows observed that, even though leaders might understand what is needed conceptually, they might lack the capacity or skills required to effect change. She asked what specific leadership capacities might be needed to reposition these organizations. Gunderson suggested that a leadership capacity that is needed is the willingness to "set our board members free" to contribute beyond the narrow definition of the role of hospital board member. He said many board members hold positions of influence across multiple organizations in different sectors (e.g., health, academia, finance). They should be able to bring all of their experiences and capacities to bear, he said. He observed that allowing bold thinking beyond defined roles is more accepted when there is a crisis to deal with, such as Ourlandia's plight, than when conditions are positive.

Bobby Milstein added that the exercise demonstrated how there is a strong tendency to operate within the boundaries of one's role. He observed that the two hospital board groups, faced with the same scenario, each tapped into a different financial resource. One sought to reposition the $45 million community health improvement funding, and the other repurposed $1 billion of the endowment. In many cases a solution depends on how the problem is framed and "the extent to which resources can be used in new ways," he said. He cautioned against "failure of imagination" and staying confined within established roles.

Meadows closed the discussion of the exercise by posing a question for participants to reflect on in their own work. "What assumptions do we have about the people we want to serve in those communities?" she asked. She suggested that the residents of a community are often not seen as assets because they are "under a dark cloud of economic and health challenges." She also charged participants to use their leadership roles in their communities to maintain the momentum in addressing these issues.

CLOSING COMMENTS

Sharfstein's perspective on the undercurrent of the day was "so close, but yet so far." He called the discussions "eye opening" and said there were many familiar and tangible approaches presented, but there was a clear gap in that these types of investments for health are not yet the norm. The challenge is how to foster more willingness on the part of health care and business investment leaders to invest for health and well-being.

Looking forward to Surgeon General Jerome Adams's forthcoming Call to Action on Community Health and Economic Prosperity, Sharfstein anticipated that it will summarize the science supporting the association between economic health and numerous public health concerns. The pathway to achieving better economic health, and thereby, improved public health, is not easy, he continued. The discussions identified some of the "bright spots" in the shift toward new value and investment in health care, but traditional thinking in health care financing persists. For the most part, health care has not moved to value-based payment models. He reflected on the suggestion by Mai Pham to redesign the physician fee schedule, and suggested that it would be very challenging to redistribute payments among the primary care providers and the subspecialists. (See Box 7-3 for a brief overview of tools and platforms for reorienting investment that were shared by several speakers.)

Sharfstein said he particularly appreciated the discussions of the values and priorities of business investors, as he was unfamiliar with that perspective. He noted his interest in the concept of the community development fund, which leverages multiple sources of capital for local

---

BOX 7-3
Workshop Highlights of Tools and Platforms Used to Establish New Concepts of Value and New Investment Priorities

This box is a collection of examples of tools and platforms shared by presenters in the course of the workshop.

Health Sector
- Anchor institution strategy (e.g., hire, buy, and live local) (Gartland)
- New Markets Tax Credits as a tool for hospital capital project, application premised on implementing anchor strategy (DePompei)
- Health care payment approach: Redesign of physician fee schedule (Pham)
- Health systems, payers, and others could pool resources for longer-term investments in community health (Knickman) and that could include local government and philanthropy (Pham); example of latter is Vickrey-Clarke-Groves mechanism for allocating shared resources[a] (Pham)

Business Sector
- Platforms for socially responsible investing or impact investing (Richter)
  - Large investment firms are creating their own platforms for scaling impact investing, such as U.S. Trust's Socially Innovative Investing platform (Rantanen)
  - Community Development Financial Institutions, such as Local Initiatives Support Corporation (Richter)
- Antidisplacement tools: Housing funds can be paired with investment as a solution to mitigate displacement due to gentrification (Jones)

---

[a] Parkes, D. C., and J. Shneidman. 2004. Distributed implementations of Vickrey-Clarke-Groves Mechanisms. In *AAMAS 2004: Proceedings of the Third Joint Conference on Autonomous and Multiagent Systems*, July 19–24, 2004, New York City, New York, USA, Ed. IEEE Computer Society. Piscataway, NJ: IEEE, pp. 261–268. https://dash.harvard.edu/handle/1/4054438 (accessed June 23, 2021).

investment. He also expressed an appreciation for both the potential and the obstacles of this approach. For example, he acknowledged the difficulty of placing a value on the fund in a manner that private individuals would be inclined to invest in it. Sharfstein recalled the discussion by Jamie Rantanen of Bank of America regarding how investors are increasingly interested in taking ESG into account when investing. Despite this growing interest, and the many opportunities to invest for impact, he believed that more specific information would be needed to understand which investments would provide the most value and be most meaningful for health and well-being.

With regard to the small group exercise, Sharfstein said it was "daunting" to have to decide where to invest vast sums of money to be successful in promoting population health. He noted the challenges of changing behavior and getting people to think and act fundamentally differently. In closing, he called on the roundtable members to consider what concrete actions the roundtable could take (e.g., publications, engagements) to make sure that the future is not so far away.

Participant Perspectives

Mary Pittman observed that this workshop bridged many of the topics that the roundtable has covered in workshops in recent years, such as education, housing, and rethinking how health care is organized and governed. She said the most significant hurdle to any solution is getting consensus on how to redistribute funding. She suggested that some of the ideas presented should be explored further by the roundtable in a future planning session. She was also interested in hearing from board members of a health system that has reoriented their values and investment priorities to learn how they were able to think and act differently.

Tufte added that it would be helpful to hear from consumers or end users who are the intended beneficiaries of these investments. What was the impact of the fiscal policies implemented and the economic development? She noted that a common phrase on boards in North Dakota is "nothing about us without us," which she said means there must be full participation of those who will be impacted by the policies.

David Kindig agreed with Sharfstein's earlier comment that the business investment leader presentation was most interesting to him. It gave him a sense of optimism that, even if health care leadership is slow to change, the new generation of investors from families of wealth seems to be embracing different standards, such as ESG standards investing.

Kaplan reiterated his earlier comment (see Chapter 3) that existing clinical medicine guidelines offer specific actions for providers to take. In many cases, however, these actions can have limited or no effect, he said.

There are no comparable guidelines for clinicians for managing the social determinants of health, and he said there is an opportunity to make specific, evidence-based suggestions for actions that can achieve outcomes.

Marc Gourevitch was encouraged by the concept of ESG investing and the increasing interest in "spending in a socially valuable way." More discussion is needed on how best to get hospitals and the population health field more engaged in this trend.

Nina Burke from ReThink Health observed that the fields of finance and health care are both necessarily highly risk averse, but innovations continue to emerge from both sectors. She noted the importance of leaders in these sectors taking risks and continuing to innovate. She suggested that the emerging generation of leaders is more willing to take risks, but might not yet have the institutional knowledge to be fully productive. She encouraged those in current leadership roles to continue to innovate, and to also engage the next generation of leaders who are "ready to take this charge forward."

Marthe Gold lamented that a "commitment to social solidarity" is lacking in the United States at the moment. Still, she said she was encouraged that the impact investing portfolios performed better than the market. This suggests, she said, that people might choose to invest in ESG portfolios, even if only for financial reasons and not for social impact reasons. She also expressed disappointment with how disengaged her own financial advisor was with regard to impact investing, and she suggested that participants have conversations about their interests in this area with their financial advisors. She also said she planned to ask whether her employer was engaged in impact investing.

Catherine Baase reiterated her question about the transparency of decision making by portfolio managers involved in ESG investments. Do companies know when they have been selected for, or excluded from, these portfolios and why? She also observed that investment choices intended to impact health and well-being are being made with little input from those with expertise in what moves population health. She suggested that greater attention needs to be paid to how this selection is made, and that there is an opportunity now for experts in population health to partner with those who manage impact investments to more effectively invest for both health and economic prosperity.

Milstein acknowledged the range of participant comments spanning pessimism to optimism. The origin of the word "wealth" derives from "well-being," he said, and only in recent centuries has there been a separation between the generation of wealth in the marketplace and the conditions that lead to health and well-being. He said he was optimistic because the workshop discussions showed there are "major market forces that are now linking health and well-being in ways that are different than they used to be." There is growing recognition that the disconnect between wealth and well-being "is producing unacceptable risk." He reiterated the comment by Rantanen (see Chapter 6) that 68 percent of the market value of S&P 500 companies is based on intangible assets. In this new knowledge economy, corporate leaders are recognizing that being on "the wrong side of a social issue" can be very commercially damaging to a company. The question, Milstein said, is the extent to which the health sector will participate in and foster the success of this trend by, for example, informing investment choices or tracking the benefits and consequences of impact investments.

Appendix A

References

IOM (Institute of Medicine). 2014. *Applying a health lens to decision making in non-health sectors: Workshop summary.* Washington, DC: The National Academies Press.

IOM. 2015a. *Financing population health improvement: Workshop summary.* Washington, DC: The National Academies Press.

IOM. 2015b. *The role and potential of communities in population health improvement: Workshop summary.* Washington, DC: The National Academies Press.

Kindig, D. 1997. *Purchasing population health: Paying for results.* Ann Arbor, MI: University of Michigan Press.

NASEM (National Academies of Sciences, Engineering, and Medicine). 2018. *Building sustainable financing structures for population health: Insights from non-health sectors: Proceedings of a workshop.* Washington, DC: The National Academies Press.

NASEM. 2019. *Exploring tax policy to advance population health, health equity, and economic prosperity: Proceedings of a workshop.* Washington, DC: The National Academies Press.

Pham, H., and P. B. Ginsburg. 2018. Payment and delivery-system reform—The next phase. *New England Journal of Medicine* 379(17):1594–1596.

Appendix B

Workshop Agenda

Reorienting Health Care and Finance Sector Investment Priorities Toward Health and Well-Being: A Workshop

December 3, 2018

New York University (NYU) Langone Health
Farkas Auditorium
550 1st Avenue, New York, New York

WORKSHOP OBJECTIVES

Workshop presentations and discussions are expected to:

1. Reflect on the history and current state of the shift to new values and investment priorities (e.g., living wages or environmental sustainability) within two spotlight sectors: health care and business investments
2. Explore what selected organizational leaders are doing to establish new concepts of value and new investment priorities
3. Elevate leadership and partnership opportunities that could help to further the shift toward new investments that produce equitable health and well-being

8:30 am   Welcome and charge to participants

   Sanne Magnan, *HealthPartners Institute and University of Minnesota*
   (Roundtable Co-Chair)

   Marc Gourevitch, *NYU Langone Health*
   (Host)

   Bobby Milstein, *ReThink Health*
   (Planning Committee Chair)

8:45 am   Keynote Address: A Call to Action from the Surgeon General to connect health and the economy

   Introduction:
   Cathy Baase, *Michigan Health Improvement Alliance and The Dow Chemical Company*

   Speaker:
   U.S. Surgeon General Jerome Adams

9:15 am   Why and how are values and priorities changing in health care?

   Dialogue with panelists and participants

   Moderator: Sanne Magnan

   Speakers:
   Hoangmai (Mai) Pham, *Anthem*
   James Knickman, *NYU Grossman School of Medicine and NYU Wagner School of Public Service*

10:10 am   Why and how are values and priorities changing among business investors?

   Dialogue with panelists and participants

   Moderator: Lisa Richter, *Avivar Capital*

   Speakers:
   Maurice Jones, *Local Initiatives Support Corporation*
   Lisa Williams, *Goldman Sachs*

11:00 am   Break

11:15 am   Health care leader profile:
           University Hospitals, Cleveland

        Moderator: Gary Gunderson, *Wake Forest Baptist Medical Center and Stakeholder Health*

        Speakers:
        Patti DePompei, *University Hospitals Rainbow Babies & Children's Hospital*
        Heidi Gartland, *University Hospitals*

12:15 pm   Lunch *(on your own)*

1:15 pm   Business investment leader profile:
           U.S. Trust at Bank of America

        Moderator: Cathy Baase

        Speaker:
        Jamie Rantanen, *U.S. Trust at Bank of America Wealth Management*

2:00 pm   Breakout group: Responses to a predicament in Ourlandia

        Facilitator:
        Phyllis Meadows, *The Kresge Foundation*

3:00 pm   Break and reconvene

3:15 pm   Portraits of necessary leadership

        Facilitator: Phyllis Meadows

4:10 pm   Reflections on the day and closing remarks

        Joshua Sharfstein, *Bloomberg School of Public Health, Johns Hopkins University* (Roundtable Co-Chair)

4:30 pm   Adjourn

Appendix C

Biographical Sketches

Vice Admiral (VADM) Jerome Adams, M.D., M.P.H., the 20th Surgeon General of the United States, was sworn into office by Vice President Mike Pence on September 5, 2017. Dr. Adams, a board-certified anesthesiologist, served as Indiana State Health Commissioner from 2014 to 2017. Dr. Adams has bachelor's degrees in both biochemistry and psychology from the University of Maryland, Baltimore County, an M.P.H. from the University of California, Berkeley, and an M.D. from the Indiana University School of Medicine. Dr. Adams was also an associate professor of clinical anesthesia at Indiana University School of Medicine and a staff anesthesiologist at Eskenazi Health, where he was the chair of the Pharmacy and Therapeutics Committee. He has served in leadership positions at a number of professional organizations, including the American Medical Association, the Indiana State Medical Association, and the Indiana Society of Anesthesiologists. He is the immediate past chair of the Professional Diversity Committee for the American Society of Anesthesiologists.

As health commissioner, Dr. Adams presided over Indiana's efforts to deal with the state's unprecedented HIV outbreak. In this capacity, he worked directly with the Centers for Disease Control and Prevention, as well as with state and local health officials and community leaders, and brought the widest range of resources, policies, and care available to stem the epidemic affecting that community. He also helped with the successful launch of Indiana's state-based, consumer-driven alternative to Medicaid expansion and worked with the state legislature to secure more than $10 million to combat infant mortality in high-risk areas of the state.

Cathy Baase, M.D., serves as the board chair of the Michigan Health Improvement Alliance, a multi-stakeholder collaborative dedicated to improving the health of people in 14 counties of central Michigan. She is a member of the Roundtable on Population Health Improvement of the National Academies of Sciences, Engineering, and Medicine and chairs its Business Collaborative. Additionally, Dr. Baase serves on the Stakeholder Engagement Subcommittee of the Secretary's Advisory Committee on National Health Promotion and Disease Prevention Objectives for 2030. She is currently a member of the National Alliance to impact the Social Determinants of Health and serves as a senior advisor to HealthBegins, which is focused on upstream efforts in health care.

Dr. Baase recently retired from her role as the chief health officer and the global director of health services for The Dow Chemical Company, a position she held for 20 years of her 32 years with Dow. While there, she had direct responsibility for leadership and management of all Occupational Health, Epidemiology, and Health Promotion programs and staff around the world. Dr. Baase was also the key driver of the Dow Health Strategy. She served as a board member of the Partnership for Prevention for more than 10 years and the Board of Directors of the Patient-Centered Primary Care Collaborative Board for 3 years. She also served on the Robert Wood Johnson Foundation Roadmaps to Health Advisory Board, the National Quality Forum's advisory group for the Multi-Stakeholder Input on a National Priority: Improving Population Health by Working with Communities project, many committee and advisory positions with the Centers for Disease Control and Prevention (CDC), and most recently on the Public Health–Health Care Collaboration Workgroup of the Advisory Committee to the Director of CDC. She was previously a member of the Clinical Research Roundtable of the Institute of Medicine.

She is a fellow in the American College of Occupational and Environmental Medicine and a fellow in the American Academy of Family Physicians. Under her leadership, the health programs of The Dow Chemical Company were extensively recognized for their innovation and achievement around the world. Dr. Baase has received numerous awards and recognition throughout her career. In 2017, she received the highest honor in occupational and environmental medicine when she was awarded the Lifetime Achievement in Occupational and Environmental Medicine Award from the American College of Occupational and Environmental Medicine. Later that year, Dr. Baase was again recognized as a distinguished executive leader in the health field as she received the 2017 Jerry Noyce Executive Health Champion Award from the Health Enhancement Research Organization.

Dr. Baase is a distinguished communicator on the topics of health strategy, prevention, occupational health, and public health and is on the editorial staff of the *American Journal of Health Promotion*. She has co-authored more than 30 publications and received many awards for leadership in the health field.

Dr. Baase graduated from the College of Human Medicine, Michigan State University, and completed a postdoctoral fellowship in primary care faculty development. She has been board certified in family practice since completing her residency at Saginaw Cooperative Hospitals Inc., where she served as the chief resident. She graduated summa cum laude from Saginaw Valley State University with degrees in chemistry and secondary education.

Patricia M. DePompei, M.S.N., was appointed the president of University Hospitals (UH) MacDonald Women's Hospital and Rainbow Babies & Children's Hospital in 2012. UH Rainbow Babies & Children's has been a trusted leader in pediatric health care for more than 125 years, consistently ranking among the top children's hospitals in the nation. Founded in 1891, UH MacDonald Women's Hospital is 1 of only 11 full-service women's hospitals in the country and the only hospital in Ohio dedicated solely to women's health. Ms. DePompei has held a variety of positions within health care over the past 30 years, including clinical and management positions in pediatric and neonatal intensive care as well as human resources. She received her M.S.N. from Kent State University and her B.S.N. cum laude from the Medical College of Ohio at the University of Toledo; and completed the Executive Management Series in Health Care at Case Western Reserve University/Weatherhead School of Management.

Ms. DePompei has served on a number of regional and national programs related to the health and wellness of children and families. She is the 2017 chair of the American Hospital Association's Section for Maternal and Child Health Governing Council. She was the chair of the Ohio Children's Hospital Association (2017–2019) and a board member of The Center for Health Affairs in Cleveland, Ohio, and the Centers for Families and Children. She was appointed to the Ohio Children's Hospital Association national "Solutions for Patient Safety" Board in 2015 and has served in a number of local organizations, including serving as chair of the Cleveland March of Dimes "March for Babies" walk, leader of the University Hospitals of Cleveland United Way campaign, Board Member of the Centers for Families and Children and the Ronald McDonald House of Cleveland. She is an alumni of Leadership Cleveland class of 2016.

Heidi Gartland, M.H.A., is a health care executive, a community leader, and a lobbyist at University Hospitals (UH) of Cleveland, a $4 billion-plus health care system with 18 hospitals and more than 25,000 physicians and employees. She leads UH's external relations and strategy, including community relations, community benefit, corporate reinvestment, strategic economic development, government and regulatory affairs, and diversity and inclusion commitments. She advocates for UH at the federal, state, and local levels, and is an experienced leader in health care public policy.

Ms. Gartland is also a dedicated civic leader. She serves on the boards of the Trauma Centers Association of America (Washington, DC), Ohio Children's Hospital Association, Urban League of Greater Cleveland, Evergreen Cooperatives, Business Volunteers Unlimited, Positive Education Program, Cleveland Neighborhood Progress, and In Counsel With Women. Ms. Gartland is currently the chair of The Center for Health Affairs, is a member of the Enterprise Community Partners' Policy & Advocacy Advisory Group, and serves on the United Way Cuyahoga County Accountable Health Community Advisory Board, as well as the Federal Reserve Bank of Cleveland Community Advisory Board.

Previously, she chaired the boards of the Institute for Health Innovation (a $7 million foundation in Columbus), NewBridge Cleveland, the Foundation for Healthy Communities, and Voices for Ohio's Children (Columbus). She also co-chaired the 2016 United Way of Greater Cleveland campaign, the Cleveland Foundation's Economic Inclusion Management Committee, and the Infant Mortality Community Health Action Team, which is part of the Greater University Circle Initiative. In addition, she was a member of the Northeast Ohio Areawide Coordinating Agency's Advisory Committee.

Honors include election as a fellow of the American College of Healthcare Executives and as a member of the American Leadership Council for Diversity in Healthcare. In 2014, Ms. Gartland was recognized as a Health Care Hero by *Crain's Cleveland Business* and was a finalist in 2013 for the ATHENA International Leadership Award. *Inside Business* magazine profiled her advocacy leadership in 2013. Ms. Gartland completed her undergraduate degree at The College of Wooster (Ohio). She earned a master's of Health Administration at The Ohio State University and a certificate in diversity management from Georgetown University. Ms. Gartland is also an adjunct faculty member teaching health policy and law in the M.B.A. program of Baldwin Wallace University and teaching the certificate in diversity management for the American Hospital Association.

Gary R. Gunderson, M.Div., D.Min., D.Div., is the vice president for faith and health, a professor of public health sciences, and (at the Divinity School) a professor of religion and the health of the public, Wake Forest Baptist Medical Center and Wake Forest University School of Divinity. He holds an undergraduate degree from Wake Forest University in History, a master's of Divinity at Emory University (with an honors thesis on economics, faith, and the hungry), and a Doctor of Ministry from the Interdenominational Theological Center in Atlanta (with a thesis on boundary leadership). He is interested in organizational and community change and how people influence complex human systems to morph in the direction of greater vitality, decency, and maybe even justice. He has always been interested in what faith has to do with any of this. It has been a curious life path, but has led through about 8 years at The Carter Center, where many of these ideas were developed, and the Rollins School of Public Health at Emory University, then 7 years as a senior executive at Methodist Le Bonheur Healthcare (a $1.5 billion faith-based hospital system in Memphis, Tennessee, one of the poorest cities in the United States). His current work focuses on helping this large system align its full institutional and human assets with its professed goal of advancing the health of the region.

Maurice A. Jones, J.D., M.S., became the fourth president and the chief executive officer of the Local Initiatives Support Corporation (LISC) in 2016. Prior to joining LISC, he served as the secretary of commerce for the Commonwealth of Virginia, where he managed 13 state agencies focused on the economic needs in his native state. He previously served as the deputy secretary for the Department of Housing and Urban Development, overseeing operations for the agency and its 8,900 staff members. Earlier, he was the commissioner of Virginia's Department of Social Services and the deputy chief of staff to former Virginia Governor Mark Warner.

Trained as an attorney, Mr. Jones worked during the Clinton administration on legal, policy, and program issues at the Department of the Treasury, where he also helped manage a then-new initiative called the Community Development Financial Institutions Fund—a federal program that has grown to be a critical supporter of nonprofits that leverage capital to bolster their communities. In the private sector, Mr. Jones was the general manager of *The Virginian-Pilot* in Norfolk and went on to become the president and the publisher of its parent company. He also worked for a Richmond law firm and a private philanthropy investing in community-based efforts to benefit children in Washington, DC.

Mr. Jones did his undergraduate work at Hampden-Sydney College, where he graduated Phi Beta Kappa and was selected as a Rhodes Scholar. At Oxford University, he earned a master's degree in international relations. He earned his J.D. from the University of Virginia School of Law.

James Knickman, Ph.D., is the Derzon Clinical Professor at the New York University (NYU) Robert F. Wagner Graduate School of Public Service. Dr. Knickman serves as the director of the Health Evaluation and Analytics Lab, a joint initiative of the Wagner Health Policy and Management Program and the NYU Grossman School of Medicine's Department of Population Health. He also has a faculty appointment at the NYU Grossman School of Medicine.

Dr. Knickman was previously the president and the chief executive officer of the New York State Health Foundation, a position he held since 2006. The Foundation focuses on high-impact interventions to bring about measurable improvements in New York's health system. Prior to that appointment, Dr. Knickman was the vice president for research and evaluation at the Robert Wood Johnson Foundation (RWJF). At RWJF, Dr. Knickman served on the executive group that set strategy and made decisions related to a $400 million annual grant-making agenda, with specific duties focused on management of grant making in the research and evaluation areas comprising approximately 25 percent of the foundation's activities. Prior to RWJF, he was professor of health policy and health administration at NYU Wagner.

Dr. Knickman serves as a board member of the National Council on Aging in Washington, DC, and of Philanthropy New York. He is a member of Fordham University's Board of Visitors, the national advisory committee of the National Resource Center for Participant-Directed Services, and the external advisory committee of the Rutgers Center for State Health Policy. He has published extensive research on issues related to the financing of health care and long-term care and improving services for frail elders, homeless families, and individuals with HIV. Dr. Knickman is the co-author of a widely used textbook on health policy and management. Dr. Knickman received a B.A. in sociology and psychology from Fordham University and a Ph.D. in public policy analysis from the University of Pennsylvania.

Sanne Magnan, M.D., Ph.D., is the co-chair of the Roundtable on Population Health Improvement of the National Academies of Sciences, Engineering, and Medicine. She is the former president and the chief executive officer of the Institute for Clinical Systems Improvement (2006–2007, 2011–2016). In 2007, she was appointed the commissioner of the Minnesota Department of Health by Minnesota Governor Tim Pawlenty. She served from 2007 to 2010 and had significant responsibility for implementation of Minnesota's 2008 health reform legislation, including the Statewide Health Improvement Program, standardized quality reporting, development of provider peer grouping, certification process for health care homes, and baskets of care.

Dr. Magnan was a staff physician at the Tuberculosis Clinic at St. Paul–Ramsey County Department of Public Health (2002–2015). She was a member of the Population-Based Payment Model Workgroup of the Healthcare Payment Learning and Action Network (2015–2016) and a member of the Centers for Medicare & Medicaid Services Multi-Sector

Collaboration Measure Development Technical Expert Panel (2016). She is on Epic's Population Health Steering Board and on the Healthy People 2030 Engagement Subcommittee.

She served on the board of MN Community Measurement and the board of NorthPoint Health & Wellness Center, a federally qualified health center and part of Hennepin Health. Her previous experience also includes vice president and medical director of consumer health at Blue Cross and Blue Shield of Minnesota. Currently, she is a senior fellow with HealthPartners Institute and an adjunct assistant professor of medicine at the University of Minnesota. Dr. Magnan holds an M.D. and a Ph.D. in medicinal chemistry from the University of Minnesota and is a board-certified internist.

Phyllis Meadows, Ph.D., R.N., M.S.N., is a senior fellow in the Health Program at The Kresge Foundation. Since joining the Foundation in 2009, she has advised the health team on the development of its overall strategic direction and provided leadership in the design and implementation of grantmaking initiatives and projects. Dr. Meadows has also coached team members and created linkages to national organizations and experts in the health field. In addition, she regularly reviews grant proposals, aids prospective grantees in preparing funding requests, and provides health-related expertise. Dr. Meadows has led the Foundation's Emerging Leaders and Public Health Program, and advises and supports the development of cross-team programming efforts with the Detroit, Environment and Human Services programs.

Dr. Meadows's 30-year career spans the nursing, public health, academic, and philanthropic sectors. She is the former associate dean for practice at the University of Michigan School of Public Health and a clinical professor in health management and policy, where she designed and implemented community-based health strategies, evaluation, research, and courses on leadership, policy, population health, and health equity. Dr. Meadows's work in public health includes serving as the deputy director and then director/public health officer for the city of Detroit. In addition to serving as adjunct faculty with the Wayne State University College of Nursing and Oakland University's School of Nursing, Dr. Meadows's professional experience includes leadership roles across the health sector, working to deliver programs and services with an array of multi-disciplinary professionals in health, education, and human services. Dr. Meadows was selected for the Kellogg International Leadership Program–Group I. After completing the three-year fellowship, she joined the W.K. Kellogg Foundation as a program director working to advance quality programs for children and youth in education and higher education, and communities nationally and internationally. She maintains an active advisory role on several national, statewide initiatives and boards that focus on improving the health of marginalized and low-income communities.

Bobby Milstein, Ph.D., M.P.H., is a director of ReThink Health for The Rippel Foundation and a visiting scientist at the Massachusetts Institute of Technology Sloan School of Management. With an educational background that combines cultural anthropology, behavioral science, and systems science, Dr. Milstein concentrates on challenges that involve large-scale institutional change and the need to align multiple lines of action. He led the development of the ReThink Health Dynamics model and a suite of regionally configured simulations that are used by leaders across the country to explore the likely health and economic consequences of policy scenarios. From 1991 to 2011, Dr. Milstein worked at the Centers for Disease Control and Prevention (CDC), where he founded the Syndemics Prevention Network, chaired the agency's Behavioral and Social Science Working Group, and was the coordinator for a wide range of new initiatives. He was the principal architect of CDC's framework for program evaluation and published a monograph titled *Hygeia's Constellation: Navigating Health Futures in a Dynamic and Democratic World*. He has led several award-winning teams that bring greater structure, evidence, and creativity to the challenge of health system change. He is a co-founder (with Patty Mabry) of the National Institutes of Health Institute on Systems Science and Health and a co-developer of several other widely used health policy simulation models, including HealthBound and the Prevention Impacts Simulation Model. He has received CDC's Honor Award for Excellence in Innovation and the Applied Systems Thinking Prize from the Applied Systems Thinking Institute, as well as Article of the Year awards from AcademyHealth and the Society for Public Health Education. Dr. Milstein holds a B.A. in cultural anthropology from the University of Michigan, an M.P.H. from Emory University, and a Ph.D. in interdisciplinary arts and sciences, with a specialization in public health science from Union Institute & University.

Hoangmai (Mai) Pham, M.D., M.P.H., is the vice president, Provider Alignment Solutions, at Anthem. She is responsible for developing and refining Anthem's provider payment models that reduce the cost of care while rewarding improvements in quality and access. Additionally, she is focused on developing new products and networks built on a foundation of value-based care, and overseeing Anthem's Enhanced Personal Health Care initiative, a program that focuses on patient-centered care and reimburses doctors for value-based, rather than volume-based, performance.

Prior to joining Anthem in 2017, Dr. Pham was a founding official at the Center for Medicare & Medicaid Innovation (CMMI), where she served as the chief innovation officer. She was responsible for the implementation of the alternative payment model provisions of the Medicare Access and Children's Health Insurance Program Reauthorization Act and other multi-organizational initiatives for the center. Her earlier work at CMMI included responsibility as the director of the Seamless Care Models Groups, overseeing the design and testing of models on accountable care organizations (ACOs) and advanced primary care, including the Pioneer and Next Generation ACO Models and Comprehensive Primary Care Initiative. Previously, she was the senior health researcher and the co-director of research at the Center for Studying Health System Change and its affiliate, Mathematica, an independent health policy organization.

As a general internist, Dr. Pham has published extensively on payment policy issues, including care fragmentation and coordination, and also practiced for several years at safety net clinics in the Washington, DC, area. She received her undergraduate degree from Harvard University, her M.D. from Temple University, and her M.P.H. from Johns Hopkins University, where she was also a Robert Wood Johnson Foundation Clinical Scholar.

Jamie Rantanen is a senior vice president and an institutional client advisor with U.S. Trust at Bank of America Private Wealth Management, in Philadelphia, Pennsylvania. Mr. Rantanen works closely with regional and national private, nonprofit, and institutional clients to distill their financial needs and objectives, pursuing those priorities with efficiency across the U.S. Trust and Bank of America platforms.

Mr. Rantanen believes strongly in helping clients understand the "impact" of their investments relative to their values and concerns. He is also adept in incorporating environmental, social, and governance (ESG) thematic investing within customized programs that identify risk and return opportunities across asset classes, as well as social and environmental impacts and outcomes.

He has extensive experience consulting to entrepreneurs, high net-worth clients and family offices, endowments and foundations, nonprofit organizations, and large institutions. Prior to joining U.S. Trust, he was head of ESG and Sustainable Investments at Deutsche Bank Asset Management, Americas. In this capacity, he led the development and implementation of the firm's ESG and strategic Sustainable Investing initiatives in the United States and served as its primary representative to clients, the marketplace, and media. For the past 17 years, he led private wealth management teams at Deutsche Bank and UBS, both in Philadelphia. He began his wealth management career in 1998 at Smith Barney after 3 years in its Institutional Equity division.

Lisa Richter, M.B.A., is a managing partner and the co-founder of Avivar Capital. Previously, Ms. Richter co-founded and led GPS Capital Partners, a national consultancy that assisted foundations and other institutions in designing and executing impact investing strategies. She co-leads Avivar's overall business activities, bringing more than two decades of fund management and investing experience spanning asset classes, return expectations, geographies and issue areas, and frequently incorporating place-based or sector focus to increase equitable access to opportunity. Clients range from small to the nation's largest independent and community foundations, banks, and institutional investors, with interests ranging from place-based outcomes to theme-based strategies that apply traditional asset allocations to earn market-rate expected returns. She authored *Grantmakers in Health Guide to Impact Investing*, co-authored *Equity Advancing Equity* (a guide to community foundation impact investing), and co-authored a rural community foundation impact investing guide. She co-designed the Mission Investors Exchange, where she continues as a lead trainer. Through early 2006, Ms. Richter led the National Community Investment Fund, a national Community Development Financial Institution (CDFI) that places equity and debt in development banking institutions and built its national network of development banks and credit unions that increase asset-building credit and financial services. Prior to that, she assisted foundation, bank, government, and community-based clients in creating or expanding development financing initiatives in urban, rural, and tribal communities throughout the United States. Ms. Richter is a senior fellow with The Philanthropic Initiative, and serves or has served as a director or an advisor to the Center for Community Development Investments of the Federal Reserve Bank of San Francisco (where she currently also serves as a scholar-in-residence), Bank of America National Community Advisory Council, Dignity Health's Community Economic Initiatives Subcommittee, *American Journal of Preventive Medicine*, CDFI Coalition, Chicago Community Loan Fund, U.S. Forum for Sustainable and Responsible Investment, and New Markets Tax Credit Coalition. She holds a B.A. and an M.B.A. from the University of Chicago. She is an adjunct instructor co-teaching a graduate course on impact investing at the University of Southern California.

Joshua M. Sharfstein, M.D., the co-chair of the Roundtable on Population Health Improvement of the National Academies of Sciences, Engineering, and Medicine, is the vice dean for public health practice and community engagement and a professor of the practice in health policy and management at the Johns Hopkins Bloomberg School of Public Health. He is also the director of the Bloomberg American Health Initiative. His book, *Public Health Crisis Survival Guide: Leadership and Management in Trying Times*, was published in May 2018 by Oxford University Press.

Previously, Dr. Sharfstein served as the secretary of the Maryland Department of Health & Mental Hygiene from 2011 to 2014. In this position, he led efforts to align Maryland's health care system with improved health outcomes, culminating in the adoption of a revised payment model for all hospital care for Maryland residents. He also oversaw the development of a statewide health improvement process with 18 local public–private coalitions and the reshaping of the state's approach to health information exchange, long-term care, and behavioral health. From 2009 to 2011, Dr. Sharfstein served as the principal deputy commissioner of the Food and Drug Administration, where he oversaw the agency's successful performance management and transparency initiatives. From 2005 to 2009, as the commissioner of health for Baltimore City, Dr. Sharfstein led innovative efforts that contributed to major declines in both overdose deaths and infant mortality rates. From 2001 to 2005, as minority professional staff and the health policy advisor for Representative Henry A. Waxman, Dr. Sharfstein was engaged in a wide range of oversight and legislative activities on health care topics, including emergency preparedness, HIV, and the politicization of science.

Dr. Sharfstein graduated summa cum laude with an A.B. in social studies from Harvard College. From 1991 to 1992, he worked on public health projects in Guatemala and Costa Rica with a Frederick Sheldon Traveling Fellowship. He graduated from Harvard Medical School, the Boston Combined Residency Program in Pediatrics at Boston Medical Center and Children's Hospital, and the fellowship in general academic pediatrics at the Boston University School of Medicine. Dr. Sharfstein was elected as a fellow of the National Academy of Medicine (2014) and the National Academy of Public Administration (2013). He serves on the Board of Population Health and Public Health Practice of the Health and Medicine Division of the National Academies and on the editorial board of the *Journal of the American Medical Association*. His awards include the Jay S. Drotman Memorial Award from the American Public Health Association (1994), Public Official of the Year from *Governing Magazine* (2008), and the Circle of Commendation Award from the Consumer Product Safety Commission (2013).

Lisa Williams, M.B.A., is a vice president in the Alternative Investments & Manager Selection (AIMS) Group, based in New York, where she is a member of AIMS Imprint. Previously, she worked at Imprint Capital, an impact investment advisory firm, where she conducted due diligence across multiple asset classes, including liquid investments, private equity, and direct debt. Prior to Imprint, she worked with Jalia Ventures, a fund focused on businesses with deep community impact, and was an associate at Citigroup in the Investment Research Division. Ms. Williams received a B.A. in business administration from Saint Peter's University and an M.B.A. from Columbia Business School, where she was a Robert Toigo Fellow.

Appendix D

Readings and Resources

NOTES: These select readings and resources are intended to provide a sampling of the rich material available on the workshop topics. Unless otherwise stated, all links accessed December 2, 2018.

REFERENCES FROM THE COMMISSIONED INFOGRAPHIC (APPENDIX E)

CBO (Congressional Budget Office). 2016. *The richest 10% hold 76% of the wealth.* https://www.cbo.gov/publication/51846.

Costanza, R., I. Kubiszweski, E. Giovannini, H. Lovins, J. McGlade, K. E. Pickett, K. Vala Ragnardottir, D. Roberts, R. De Vogli, and R. Wilkinson. 2014. GDP and Life Satisfaction are not closely correlated. *Nature* 505(7483). https://www.nature.com/news/development-time-to-leave-gdp-behind-1.14499.

Cuckler, G. A., A. M. Sisko, J. A. Poisal, S. P. Keehan, S. D. Smith, A. J. Madison, C. J. Wolfe, and J. C. Hardesty. 2017. Healthcare spending in 2026 is projected to be $5.7T. *Health Affairs* 37(3):482–492. https://www.healthaffairs.org/doi/abs/10.1377/hlthaff.2017.1655. [Cited as CMS, 2017, in infographic.]

OECD (Organisation for Economic Co-operation and Development). 2017. *Healthcare costs in the US are 2.5X other OECD countries.* https://www.oecd-ilibrary.org/social-issues-migration-health/health-at-a-glance-2017_health_glance-2017-en;jsessionid=-9WQSaummIhZSexDdOk13tePH.ip-10-240-5-4.

Planned Giving Design Center. 2011. *A new generation of investors is likely to inherit $40T.* https://www.pgdc.com/pgdc/why-41-trillion-wealth-transfer-estimate-still-valid.

SELECTED READINGS FROM THE FIELD OF HEALTH CARE AND POPULATION HEALTH

Changing Concepts of Value and Payment Reform

AcademyHealth. 2017. *Bridging the divide: Supplementing payment reform to promote needed investments in population health.* https://www.academyhealth.org/blog/2017-04/bridging-divide-supplementing-payment-reform-promote-needed-investments-population.

AcademyHealth. n.d. *Payment reform publications.* https://www.academyhealth.org/about/programs/payment-reform-population-health.

Ash, A. S., E. O. Mick, R. P. Ellis, C. I. Kiefe, J. J. Allison, and M. A. Clark. 2017. Social determinants of health in managed care payment formulas. *JAMA Internal Medicine* 177(10):1424–1430.

Graber, D. R., and A. O. Kilpatrick. 2008. Establishing values-based leadership and value systems in healthcare organizations. *Journal of Health and Human Services Administration* 31(2):179–197.

Homer, J., B. Milstein, G. Hirsch, and E. Fisher. 2016. Combined regional investments could substantially enhance health system performance and be financially affordable. *Health Affairs* 35(8):1435–1443.

Kindig, D. A. 1997. *Purchasing population health: Paying for results.* Ann Arbor, MI: University of Michigan Press.

Kindig, D. 2015. From health determinant benchmarks to health investment benchmarks. *Preventing Chronic Disease* 12:1500–1510.

Magnan, S. J., and D. A. Kindig. 2018. Purchasing population health—revisited. *Population Health Management* 22(2):91–92.

Muhlestein, D., R. Saunders, R. Richards, and M. McClellan. 2018. Recent progress in the value journey: Growth of ACOs and value-based payment models. *Health Affairs Blog.* https://www.healthaffairs.org/do/10.1377/hblog20180810.481968/full.

Murray, R., A. E. Caballero, and S. F. Delbanco. 2018. The state of the evidence on payment reform. *NEJM Catalyst.* https://catalyst.nejm.org/state-evidence-payment-reform-shared-savings.

New York University Langone Health. 2018. Drivers of hospital investment in community health. *Learning Center on Enhancing the Role of Hospitals in Improving Public Health.* https://med.nyu.edu/chids/projects/enhancing-role-hospitals-improving-public-health.

Pham, H., and P. B. Ginsburg. 2018. Payment and delivery-system reform—The next phase. *New England Journal of Medicine* 379(17):1594–1596.

Population-based Payment Work Group. 2016. Accelerating and aligning population-based payment models: Performance measurement. *Health Care Payment Learning and Action Network.* https://hcp-lan.org/workproducts/pm-whitepaper-final.pdf.

Sharfstein, J. M., S. Gerovich, and D. Chin. 2017. Global budgets for safety-net hospitals. *JAMA* 318(18):1759–1760.

Shortell, S. M. 2013. A bold proposal for advancing population health. *NAM Perspectives.* Discussion Paper, National Academy of Medicine, Washington, DC. https://nam.edu/perspectives-2013-a-bold-proposal-for-advancing-population-health.

Song, Z., and E. S. Fisher. 2016. The ACO experiment in infancy—looking back and looking forward. *JAMA* 316(7):705–706.

Changing Accountabilities

AcademyHealth. 2017. Striving toward a culture of health: How do care and costs for non-medical needs get factored into alternative payment models. *Workshop summary & lessons learned.* https://www.academyhealth.org/sites/default/files/FINAL.AH_RWJF_Report_Striving_toward_culture_of_health.pdf.

AcademyHealth. 2018a. *Approaches to cross-sector population health accountability.* https://www.academyhealth.org/sites/default/files/Approaches_to_CrossSector_Pop_Health_Jan2018_0.pdf.

AcademyHealth. 2018b. *Striving toward a culture of health: How regional collaboratives can advance funding and financing to improve population health.* https://www.academyhealth.org/sites/default/files/regional_collaboratives_financing_pop_health_feb2018.pdf.
Includes
- A: Multi-Stakeholder Governance for Population Health: A list of key attributes for the governance of successful multi-stakeholder regional collaboratives to improve the financing and implementation of population health.
- B: Community-Based Population Health Payment Reform Readiness Assessment Tool

Mongeon, M., J. Levi, and J. Heinrich. 2017. Elements of accountable communities for health: A review of the literature. *NAM Perspectives.* Discussion Paper, National Academy of Medicine, Washington, DC. https://nam.edu/elements-of-accountable-communities-for-health-a-review-of-the-literature.

Siegel, B., J. Erickson, B. Milstein, and K. E. Pritchard. 2018. Multisector partnerships need further development to fulfill aspirations for transforming regional health and well-being. *Health Affairs* 37(1):30–37.

Anchor Roles and Organizational Case Studies (on investments, framing of value, etc.)

Democracy Collaborative. 2017. Rush University Medical Center. *The Anchor Mission playbook.* https://democracycollaborative.org/content/anchor-mission-playbook.

Martin, N. 2017. *Advancing the anchor mission of healthcare.* https://democracycollaborative.org/content/advancing-anchor-mission-healthcare-report.

Norris, T., and T. Howard. 2015. *Can hospitals heal America's communities?* Democracy Collaborative. https://democracycollaborative.org/content/can-hospitals-heal-americas-communities-0.

Oostra, R. 2018. *Embracing an anchor mission: ProMedica's all-in strategy.* Democracy Collaborative. https://democracycollaborative.org/content/embracing-anchor-mission-promedica-s-all-strategy.

Zuckerman, D. 2013a. *Hospitals building healthier communities: Embracing the anchor mission.* Democracy Collaborative. https://democracycollaborative.org/content/hospitals-building-healthier-communities-embracing-anchor-mission.

Zuckerman, D. 2013b. *Case study: Henry Ford Health System (Detroit, MI).* Democracy Collaborative. https://democracycollaborative.org/content/case-study-henry-ford-health-system-detroit-mi.

Zuckerman, D., and K. Parker. 2016a. *Hospitals aligned for healthy communities: Inclusive, local sourcing.* Democracy Collaborative. https://democracycollaborative.org/content/hospitals-aligned-healthy-communities-inclusive-local-sourcing.

Zuckerman, D., and K. Parker. 2016b. *Hospitals aligned for healthy communities: Place-based investing.* Democracy Collaborative. https://democracycollaborative.org/content/hospitals-aligned-healthy-communities-place-based-investing.

Zuckerman, D., and K. Parker. 2016c. *Hospitals aligned for healthy communities: Inclusive, local hiring.* Democracy Collaborative. https://democracycollaborative.org/content/hospitals-aligned-healthy-communities-inclusive-local-hiring.

SELECTED READINGS FROM THE FIELD OF BUSINESS INVESTMENT

Socially Responsible Impact Investing

Balboni, E., and C. Travers. 2017. *CDFIs and impact investing: An industry review.* Local Initiatives Support Corporation. http://www.lisc.org/our-resources/resource/cdfis-impact-investing-industry-review.

Democracy Collaborative. 2017. *The role of impact investors in taking employee ownership to scale.* https://democracycollaborative.org/content/role-impact-investors-taking-employee-ownership-scale.

Emerson, J. 2018a. The politics of impact. *Stanford Social Innovation Review.* https://ssir.org/book_reviews/entry/the_politics_of_impact.

Emerson, J. 2018b. *The purpose of capital: Elements of impact, financial flows, and natural being.* San Francisco, CA: Blended Value Group Press. https://www.purposeofcapital.org.

Federal Reserve Bank of San Francisco. 2012. *Investing in what works for America's communities.* http://www.whatworksforamerica.org/ideas-that-work.

Federal Reserve Bank of San Francisco. 2017. *What matters: Investing in results to build strong communities.* http://investinresults.org/book.

Global Impact Investing Network. *What you need to know about impact investing.* https://thegiin.org/impact-investing/need-to-know.

Global Impact Investing Network. *Roadmap for the future of impact investing: Reshaping financial markets.* https://thegiin.org/research/publication/giin-roadmap.

Grantmakers in Health. *Guide to impact investing.* www.gih.org/Publications/StrategicDetail.cfm?itemnumber=4097.

Kell, G. 2018. The future of corporate responsibility. *Forbes.* https://www.forbes.com/sites/georgkell/2018/06/18/the-future-of-corporate-responsibility/#c6a0256105ee.

Millay, T. 2016. Social investing: The good, the bad, and the ugly. *Forbes.* https://www.forbes.com/sites/toddmillay/2016/02/29/social-investing-the-good-the-bad-and-the-ugly/#70d1dcc98ba0.

Statler, K. 2018. Socially responsible investing delivers: Fortunately, there's no need to sacrifice performance while also doing good. *U.S. News & World Report.* https://money.usnews.com/money/blogs/the-smarter-mutual-fund-investor/articles/2018-06-07/socially-responsible-investing-delivers-for-investors.

Walkate, H., and C. Krosinsky. 2018. A more enlightened approach to SDG investing. *Stanford Social Innovation Review.* https://ssir.org/articles/entry/a_more_enlightened_approach_to_sdg_investing.

New Concepts of Value, New Ways to Invest, Transition to a Well-Being Economy

Case-Ruchala, D. 2018. *A next system of community investment: Community Reinvestment Act reform in the 21st century.* The Next System Project, Democracy Collaborative. https://thenextsystem.org/learn/stories/cra-reform?mc_cid=aa82d3d47c&mc_eid=77b8e17464.

Coalition for Inclusive Capitalism. 2018. *EPIC: Embankment Project for Inclusive Capitalism.* https://www.epic-value.com/#report.

Gordon, C. *Growing apart: A political history of American inequality.* http://scalar.usc.edu/works/growing-apart-a-political-history-of-american-inequality/index.

Green, T. 2018. What a society designed for well-being looks like. *Yes Magazine.* https://www.yesmagazine.org/issues/mental-health/what-a-society-design-for-well-being-looks-like-20180912.

Jones, M. 2017. *LISC pledges new commitment to health.* Local Initiatives Support Corporation. http://www.lisc.org/our-stories/story/lisc-pledges-new-commitment-health.

JUST Capital. 2018. *Not just another survey: JUST Capital's roadmap for corporate America.* https://justcapital.com/news/roadmap-for-corporate-america.

Leonhardt, D. 2017. Our broken economy in one simple chart. Op-Ed. *The New York Times.* https://www.nytimes.com/interactive/2017/08/07/opinion/leonhardt-income-inequality.html.

Leonhardt, D. 2018. We're measuring the economy all wrong. Op-Ed. *The New York Times.* https://nyti.ms/2N8AcDj.

Wellbeing Economy Alliance. *Understanding the wellbeing economy: Resource library.* https://wellbeingeconomy.org/resources.

Management of Common Resources

Department of Health and Human Services' Office of the Assistant Secretary for Health. 2018. *Healthy People 2030 framework.* Prepared by the Secretary's Advisory Committee on National Health Promotion and Disease Prevention Objectives for 2030. https://www.healthypeople.gov/2020/About-Healthy-People/Development-Healthy-People-2030/Framework.

Federal Reserve Bank of San Francisco. 2018. What is racial equity? *SF Fed Blog.* https://www.frbsf.org/our-district/about/sf-fed-blog/what-is-racial-equity.

IOM (Institute of Medicine). 2013. *For the public's health: Investing in a healthier future.* Washington, DC: The National Academies Press. https://www.nap.edu/catalog/13268.

Nichols, L. M., and L. A. Taylor. 2018. Social determinants as public goods: A new approach to financing key investments in healthy communities. *Health Affairs* 37(8):1223–1230.

Ostrom, E. 2009. *Beyond markets and states: Polycentric governance of complex economic systems.* Stockholm, Sweden: Nobel Prize Lecture. http://www.nobelprize.org/nobel_prizes/economic-sciences/laureates/2009/ostrom-lecture.html.

SELECTED GRAPHICS

Coalition for Inclusive Capitalism. 2018. *EPIC: Embankment Project for Inclusive Capitalism.* https://www.epic-value.com/#report. (Figure from page 13 illustrating short- and long-term value perspectives.)

United Nations Development Programme. 2016. *Sustainable development goals.* http://www.undp.org/content/dam/undp/library/corporate/brochure/SDGs_Booklet_Web_En.pdf. (Figure from page 2 of brochure.)

Appendix E

Commissioned Infographic: Path Toward a Well-Being Economy

This infographic was developed by Bobby Milstein and Sara Ivey to serve as a resource and point of reference for the workshop. The worksheet for the small group exercise was developed by Bobby Milstein with assistance from the roundtable staff.

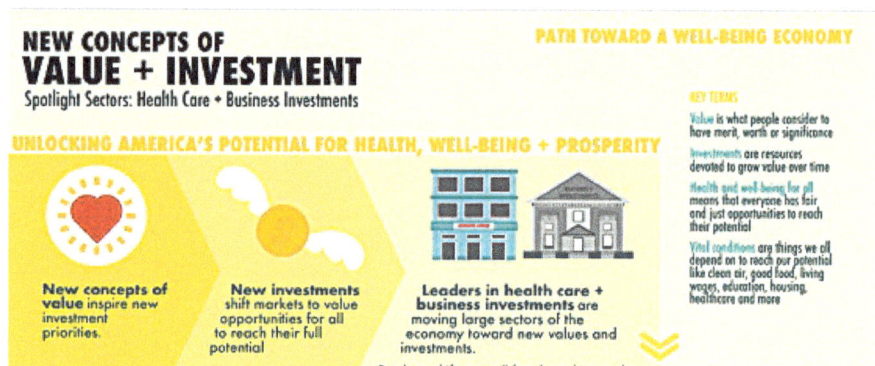

A WORKSHOP ON
Reorienting Health Care and Business Investment Priorities Toward Health and Well-Being

New York City - December 3, 2018

This graphic was created by Sara Ivey and Bobby Milstein, with support from the Roundtable on Population Health Improvement, to inform discussion at the workshop on "Reorienting Health Care and Business Investment Priorities Toward Health and Well-being Roundtable." The authors are responsible for the content of this graphic which does not necessarily reflect the views of the National Academies of Sciences, Engineering, and Medicine or the Roundtable on Population Health Improvement.

GO TO WORKSHOP MATERIALS

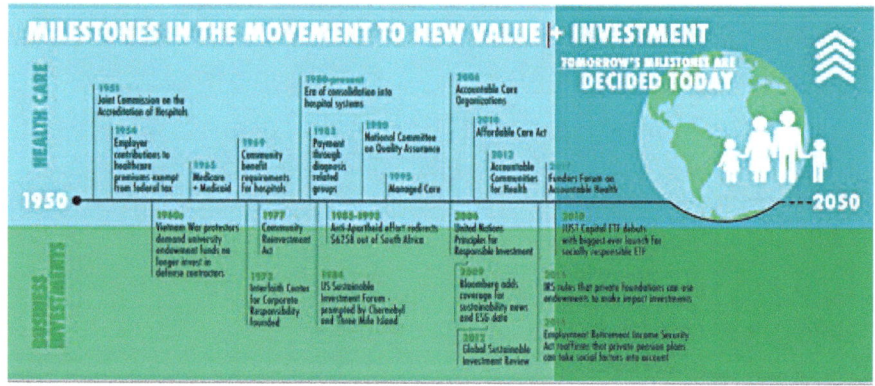

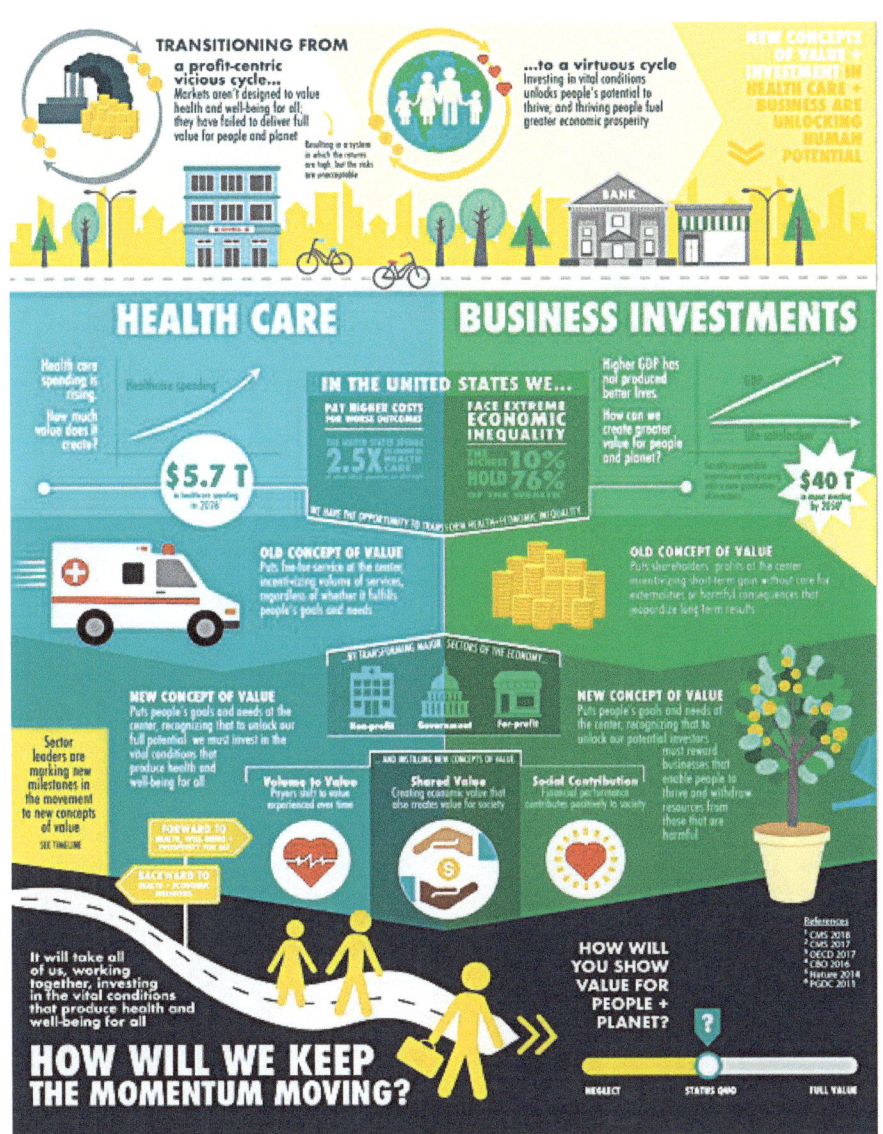

Appendix F

Small Group Exercise Materials

Following the panel discussions, workshop participants broke into small groups to discuss investment priorities for health and well-being, as well as organizational and leadership challenges, for the fictional city of Ourlandia.

NASEM Roundtable on Population Health Improvement
Workshop on Reorienting Health Care and Business Investments Toward Health and Well-Being

The Predicament

- Ourlandia is a mid-sized American city, once the nation's leading manufacturer of industrial glass; it is also a regional hub for telecommunications, agriculture, higher education, and vocational training. Nearby lakes and forests attract tourism, service industries, and artists.
- Fortunes in the glass industry declined along with all US manufacturing. City leaders were slow to plan for socio-economic transition.
- Population declined 15% in 30 years, and will fall more without a rebound plan.
- Residents include a mix of classes and cultures, all immersed in a long, painful history of residential segregation, concentrated poverty, white flight, suburban sprawl, extreme wealth inequality, disrespect for indigenous people, and denial of full human dignity for women, people of color, and other subgroups.
- People and the economy suffer from excessively high and inequitable rates of chronic illness, addiction, suicide, violence, poverty, and unjust incarceration. Wildfires have been intensifying, along with eroding air and water quality.
- Life expectancy has fallen for the past three years.
- More than 60% believe the next generation will live worse lives than their parents.

Civic Assets
- Inclusive values and pioneering spirit
- Pragmatic people willing to work across differences to respond to common problems or injustice
- Trusted leaders and organized residents

Your Charge: Participate in the renaissance of Ourlandia

Background in Spotlight Sectors

Health Care	Business Investment
• Ourlandia's main nonprofit hospital was built in 1908 by wealthy industrialists and Catholic nuns as a free clinic for factory families.	• Small companies and major corporations that do business in Ourlandia are sensitive to strong public expectations regarding fair treatment of workers and customers; product safety; environmental sustainability; and ethical management.
• Over the past 40 years, two other small hospitals formed and all three eventually merged, as the health care sector became a big business unto itself. Ourlandia Hospital is now a major nonprofit center for teaching and research, the second largest employer, and an anchor of the regional economy.	• Local banks and credit unions support community development and routinely fulfill requirements of the Community Reinvestment Act. Big national banks are sometimes less compliant and have been publicly sanctioned.
• The hospital's current business model is breaking down. Most payers will end fee-for-service payment in the next decade. Half of the population is already covered through value-based contracts. There is now a strong economic incentive to not only care for acute illness, but also to sustain equitable health and well-being for as long as possible.	• A large multi-employer pension fund (supporting public and private employees) remains solvent and was among the first to adopt socially-responsible investment criteria, with a focus on living wages, gender equity, and renewable energy.

APPENDIX F

Examples of Emerging Values & Investments

Below are several early-stage initiatives that are gaining traction and need greater investment to yield their full value for health and well-being across Ourlandia. Keep in mind that past gains are also fragile and must be maintained.

Food Security	Routine Care & Resilience	Safety & Criminal Justice
Farmers, food distributors, advertisers, schools, and large employers form a joint venture to end hunger and food insecurity	Popular mind-body centers offer easy access to affordable preventive and chronic care, smoking cessation, addiction recovery, stress reduction, trauma-informed resilience, and other routine services	Bipartisan criminal justice reform creates a framework for public safety, fair treatment for nonviolent offenses, and an end of the school-to-prison pipeline
College & Wealth	**Wages & Workplaces**	**Biotech for Prevention**
Employers and public educators offer student debt waivers and free college tuition in exchange for work in a new *Community Stewardship Corps*	Consumers and hourly workers persuade employers to pay living wages, guarantee worker safety, and support sick leave, or risk boycotts and other kinds of public backlash	Engineers and biotech firms team up with glass manufacturers to design the next generation of fiber optics for diagnostic screening and high-speed computing
Ownership & Purpose	**OTHERS**	**Nature & Land Use**
Tax policies offer windfall profits to corporations that expand employee ownership or covert to B-corporations	There are many other opportunities to enhance vital conditions for health and well-being. If you don't see your highest priorities, be creative and propose something new.	Land trusts convert vacant and abandoned lots into to playspaces, gardens, and outdoor classrooms
Transportation	**Racial Equity & Social Justice**	**Multisector Accountability**
New transportation tax credits provide incentives for active transport, mass transit, remote work, and telemedicine	City Council debates an ordinance to emphasize racial equity and social justice in all policies and practices	An *Accountable Community for Ourlandia's Future* launches with 1,200+ organizations from every sector that commit to a common portfolio of effective and efficient investments
Corporate Citizenship	**Aging at Home**	**Clean Environment**
Local media begin to broadcast weekly stories of inspiring corporate citizenship—as well as scandalous examples of greed and harm	Building codes and tax policies enable seniors to remain at home and age in place	Carbon pricing and a green building fund improve cost-effectiveness for clean power, clean air and water, while lowering the cost of utilities for families and responsible businesses

How Will You Contribute to the Renaissance of Ourlandia?

Step 1: Consider Your Role

You and your fellow group members will play just one assigned role (either a Hospital Board or a Pension Fund Manager). Here is a short description of each role.

Board of Ourlandia Hospital	Pension Fund Manager
Your Role & Strategic Imperatives:	*Your Role & Strategic Imperatives:*
• Reposition the nonprofit hospital as a high-value producer of health and well-being for all, not only a place to care for acute illness/injury	• Safeguard and enhance lifelong economic security for working families, while fulfilling obligations for socially responsible investing
• Establish clear organizational values, investment priorities, and partnerships	• Establish clear organizational values, investment priorities, and partnerships
• Generate the greatest possible human and financial value through	• Generate the greatest possible human and financial value through
o Strong civic leadership	o Strong civic leadership
o 15,000 employees	o 200,000 workers and retirees
o $4.5B endowment	o $20B assets under management
o $450M annual revenues	o 20+ year time horizon
o $45M annual comm. health improvement	

Step 2: Identify Your Priorities for Value & Investment

- Review emerging opportunities, consider trade-offs, and name your priorities (15 minutes)
- Describe major changes in organizational role and leadership challenges (20 minutes)

Questions	Responses
Which are the most compelling priorities to enhance value for your organization and for Ourlandia? *Bonus: Write a short headline*	
How do these priorities reposition your role in Ourlandia?	
What trade-offs did you consider when setting your priorities?	
What leadership challenges will you have to overcome (within your organization or with others)?	